SpringerBriefs in Population Studies

SpringerBriefs in Population Studies presents concise summaries of cutting-edge research and practical applications across the field of demography and population studies. It publishes compact refereed monographs under the editorial supervision of an international Advisory Board. Volumes are compact, 50 to 125 pages, with a clear focus. The series covers a range of content from professional to academic such as: timely reports of state-of-the art analytical techniques, bridges between new research results, snapshots of hot and/or emerging topics, and in-depth case studies.

The scope of the series spans the entire field of demography and population studies, with a view to significantly advance research. The character of the series is international and multidisciplinary and includes research areas such as: population aging, fertility and family dynamics, demography, migration, population health, household structures, mortality, human geography and environment. Volumes in this series may analyze past, present and/or future trends, as well as their determinants and consequences. Both solicited and unsolicited manuscripts are considered for publication in this series.

SpringerBriefs in Population Studies will be of interest to a wide range of individuals with interests in population studies, including demographers, population geographers, sociologists, economists, political scientists, epidemiologists and health researchers as well as practitioners across the social sciences.

More information about this series at http://www.springer.com/series/10047

George B. Ploubidis · Benedetta Pongiglione ·
Bianca De Stavola · Rhian Daniel ·
Lenka Benova · Emily Grundy ·
Sanna Read

Pathways to Health

Springer

George B. Ploubidis
Centre for Longitudinal Studies
UCL Institute of Education
University College London
London, UK

Bianca De Stavola
Great Ormond Street Institute of Child Health
University College London
London, UK

Lenka Benova
Institute of Tropical Medicine
Antwerp, Belgium

Sanna Read
Personal Social Services Research Unit
London School of Economics and Political Science
London, UK

Benedetta Pongiglione
CERGAS
Bocconi University
Milano, Italy

Rhian Daniel
University of Hospital Wales
Cardiff University School of Medicine
Cardiff, UK

Emily Grundy
Institute for Social and Economic Research
University of Essex
Colchester, UK

ISSN 2211-3215 ISSN 2211-3223 (electronic)
SpringerBriefs in Population Studies
ISBN 978-94-024-1705-0 ISBN 978-94-024-1707-4 (eBook)
https://doi.org/10.1007/978-94-024-1707-4

This Springer imprint is published by the registered company Springer Nature B.V.
The registered company address is: Van Godewijckstraat 30, 3311 GX Dordrecht, The Netherlands

Preface

Health is of fundamental importance for both national and individual well-being and ill health has major implications for individuals, their families and communities, employers, service providers and society as a whole. Extensive research has shown that socio-economic and demographic factors are associated with health outcomes and the importance of these associations for public policy is widely recognised, as shown by national and international commissions on the Social Determinants of Health. For the development and assessment of strategies to improve health, it is of crucial importance to understand which pathways link social and biological disadvantage, and whether such pathways act across generations as well as within a lifetime. Recent years have seen major advances in our understanding of some of these processes, including recognition of pre-natal, early life and other life course influences on adult diseases, as well as developments in the conceptualization of the possible pathways linking socio-economic, demographic and community contexts to health. There has also been substantial advances in methodology for the study of pathways—in particular for the formal identification of mediating factors—and for dealing with ubiquitous sources of systematic bias, such as missing data and measurement error.

This book has its origins on the National Centre for Research Methods node "Pathways" that was funded by the Economic and Social Research Council between 2011 and 2014. Pathways had a substantive as well as a closely linked methodological focus which is reflected in the chapters of the current volume. The substantive focus was on the investigation of pathways that link socio-demographic circumstances to health with an emphasis on the mediating factors that lie on these pathways, while the methodological focus was in the development and dissemination of rigorous approaches for the formal identification and quantification of these pathways. The integration of methodological approaches to simultaneously deal with challenges such as measurement error and missing data in applications where pathways or other life course processes are formally quantified is the core focus of this volume.

We believe that this integration will enhance the ability of the social science community to investigate specific hypotheses and potentially inform public health interventions, and also promote methodological exchange between the social and biomedical research communities. The dissemination and facilitation of such integrated methods among the social science community is timely, given the increasing availability of individual-level data on biological and social dimensions measured over time and the complexity of the mechanisms that link these dimensions over the life course.

The four chapters presented here capitalise on the richness of UK-based longitudinal surveys that allow the investigation of complex mechanisms and the rigorous quantification of pathways to health over the life course, while simultaneously dealing with biases due to missing data and measurement error. Rhian Daniel and Bianca De Stavola in Chap. 1 provide us with a thorough but accessible introduction to the latest developments in mediation analysis which is crucial for the appropriate estimation of pathways. The authors clarify the assumptions implicit in approaches such as Structural Equation Modelling and how these are relaxed within the counterfactual approach, highlighting particular issues such as intermediate confounding which is particularly pertinent in longitudinal and life course studies. In Chap. 2, Ploubidis, Benova, De Stavola & Grundy, combine Linear Structural Equation Modelling with the parametric G formula to investigate the life course patterning of socio-economic position induced differences in health related behaviour. By formally quantifying the pathways through which socio-economic position at various stages of the life course is hypothesized to influence health-related behaviour, the authors showed socio-economic gradients in smoking, physical activity and alcohol use, but to a lesser extent in healthy dietary habits. Read & Grundy in Chap. 3 employ latent change score modelling within a Linear Structural Equation Modelling framework to investigate the role of physical activity as a moderator and/or mediator of the association between fertility history and later life health. By formally quantifying the concepts of mediation and interaction, the authors show that physical activity serves as a mediator in the association between fertility history and the level of later life functioning, but that it also moderates the level of health disadvantages related to high number of children and parenthood. In the last chapter, Ploubidis & Pongiglionne conceptualise pathways to health as life course trajectories and compare the evolution of self-rated health over the life course in two generations born 12 years apart in twentieth century Britain. They find that the evolution of self-rated health over time differed between the two cohorts, both with respect to the shape of change over time as well as the average level of reported self-rated health. They also document a worrying increase in self-reported bad health in the more recently born cohort, which given the expected increase in life expectancy, has major policy implications, given that the increase has occurred despite economic growth.

To round things off, I would like to thank the contributors of this book for their excellent and hard work. It was a great pleasure working with a multidisciplinary team during the three years of the Pathways project as well as the book. I would also like to thank the Centre for Longitudinal Studies and the Institute for Fiscal

Studies at University College London as well as their funders for making the longitudinal data used in this book freely available to all scientists worldwide via the UK Data Service.

London, UK George B. Ploubidis

Contents

About the Authors

George B. Ploubidis is Professor of Population Health and Statistics at University College London (UCL) and currently holds the posts of Director of Research and Chief Statistician at the UCL Centre for Longitudinal Studies. Prior to joining UCL, he held posts at the London School of Hygiene and Tropical Medicine and the University of Cambridge. He is a multidisciplinary Quantitative Social Scientist with a primary interest in socio-economic and demographic determinants of population health and the mechanisms that link these over the life course.

Benedetta Pongiglione holds a Ph.D. in Epidemiology and Population Health from the London School of Hygiene and Tropical Medicine, University of London. She previously obtained a degree in Economic and Social Science from Bocconi University and completed the European Doctoral School of Demography program. She is currently involved on research on cost and outcome analysis of healthcare technologies and development of scientific models to investigate medical practice variations to foster the use of economic evaluation in policymaking. Benedetta's research interests include socio-structural inequalities in health, and understanding their causes and consequences.

Bianca De Stavola joined UCL GOS Institute of Child Health after 23 years at the London School of Hygiene and Tropical Medicine where she was Professor of Biostatistics in the Department of Medical Statistics and co-Director of the Centre for Statistical Methodology. Bianca's main research activities involve the understanding, development and implementation of statistical methods for long-term longitudinal studies, with specific applications to life-course epidemiology. As these often involve causal enquiries, in particular, related to understanding pathways towards disease development, mediation analysis is her main interest.

Rhian Daniel is a statistician with a particular focus on methods for learning about cause-effect relationships from observational data. She is especially interested in situations, such as when attempting to learn about the joint effects of sequential exposures in the presence of time-dependent confounding, or when attempting to disentangle path-specific causal effects, where standard regression methods are known to be valid only under highly unrealistic assumptions, but where alternative, so-called "causal inference", methods rely on weaker assumptions and hence can deliver substantially more reliable inferences with respect to the question of scientific interest.

Lenka Benova is a quantitative population health scientist with training in management, economics, Middle East studies and demography. From 2014–2018, she served as a co-investigator on the Maternal healthcare markets Evaluation Team (MET) at the London School of Hygiene & Tropical Medicine, where she led the SAGE (Secondary data Analysis for Generating new Evidence) team. Her keen interest in health-seeking behaviour, maternal health research, and evaluation in low- and middle-income countries. Within these areas, she is interested in innovative methods to capture decisions and steps in health-seeking, validity of self-reported health-seeking indicators, and coverage of care contact and content.

Emily Grundy is Professor of Population Science and Director of the Institute of Social and Economic Research (ISER) at the University of Essex. Previous appointments have been at the London School of Economics, University of Cambridge, London School of Hygiene & Tropical Medicine and King's College, London. She is a demographer by training and most of her work has focussed on ageing. Her main research interests are families, households and kin and social networks in later life, especially in relationship to health, associations between family life courses, health and well-being at older ages, and trends and differentials in later life health, disability and mortality.

Sanna Read is an Assistant Professorial Research Fellow at the Personal Social Services Research Unit, London School of Economics and Political Science. Her current research interests are long-term health effects of fertility history, social contacts and socio-economic factors in middle and older age. She is also interested in social inequalities and school engagement, school burnout and mental health among young people.

Chapter 1
Mediation Analysis for Life Course Studies

Rhian M. Daniel and Bianca L. De Stavola

Abstract The main aim of life course epidemiology is to elucidate the processes that link early life factors to later life health. Mediation analysis plays an important role in these investigations since it offers the potential to use empirical data and statistical tools to separate the influence of an exposure on an outcome into effects through and around potential mediators. In this chapter, we have attempted to give a thorough but accessible introduction to causal mediation analysis and how it relates to Structural Equation Modelling (SEM). In particular we have reviewed the assumptions implicit in the traditional approach for the desired interpretation of mediation effects to be justified, and how many of these are relaxed when adopting the more flexible counterfactual-based approach. We have highlighted particular aspects, such as intermediate confounding and survival outcomes, which are particularly pertinent in life course investigations.

Keywords Causal mediation · Life course epidemiology · Potential outcomes

1.1 Introduction

The main aim of life course epidemiology is to elucidate the processes that link early life factors to later life health. Mediation analysis plays an important role in these investigations since it offers the potential to use empirical data and statistical tools to separate the influence of an exposure on an outcome into effects *through* and *around* potential mediators, i.e. variables (or processes) that happen between exposure and outcome.

R. M. Daniel (✉) · B. L. De Stavola (✉)
Department of Medical Statistics, Centre for Statistical Methodology, London School of Hygiene and Tropical Medicine, London, UK
e-mail: danielr8@cardiff.ac.uk

B. L. De Stavola
e-mail: b.destavola@ucl.ac.uk

G. B. Ploubidis et al., *Pathways to Health*,
SpringerBriefs in Population Studies,
https://doi.org/10.1007/978-94-024-1707-4_1

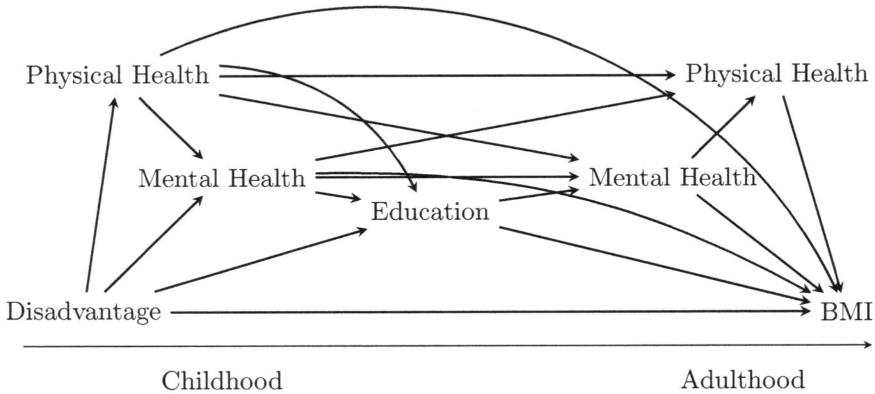

Fig. 1.1 An example taken from life course epidemiology

Consider the example shown in Fig. 1.1, where the underlying processes linking socio-economic disadvantage in childhood to body mass index (BMI) in adulthood are depicted as potentially acting through physical and mental health in childhood, educational attainment and physical health in adulthood. Given good quality data on all the variables included in this diagram (together with potential confounding variables, all to be discussed later), some form of mediation analysis could be attempted in order to estimate the strength of some or all of the various pathways from exposure to outcome. For example, we may aim to estimate how much of the effect is via the physical health pathway, how much is via mental health, and how much via education; the remainder would typically then be called the *direct* effect, not because it is direct in any absolute sense, but because it is not mediated by any of the mediators under study. Simpler enquiries could also be formulated within the mediation analysis framework; for example, we could study only the mediating role of educational achievement. The effect through education would then be the only *indirect* effect of interest, with all other path-specific effects absorbed into the direct effect.

There are two main strands in the literature dedicated to the study of mediation. The first is anchored within the social sciences where there is a strong tradition of estimating path-specific effects of an exposure using Wright's path analysis Wright (1934), later popularised by Baron and Kenny (1986) and often implemented within the framework of structural equation models (SEMs) Bollen (1989). The second strand stems from the more recent causal inference literature largely based on the potential outcomes (or counterfactual) framework (Robins, 1986; Rubin, 1974), where a more formal and general treatment of the definitions, assumptions, models and methods involved has been developed (Pearl, 2001; Robins, 1992; Vanderweele, 2015). Both approaches are being used in life course epidemiology: see (Bartoli et al., 2016; Biarnes, Arias, Alonso, & Garcia, 2015; Harris et al., 2016; Krebs et al., 2016; Kupers et al., 2015; Kushner, Quilty, Uliaszek, McBride, & Bagby, 2016; Rodgers et al., 2016; Rauscher et al., 2016; van Iersel, Kiesner, Pastore, & Scholte, 2016) for recent examples of the path analysis approach and (Benedum, Yazdy, Parker, Mitchell, & Werler, 2016; Chen, Mukherjee, Ferguson, Meeker, & VanderWeele, 2016; Jackson, VanderWeele, Blacker, & Schneeweiss, 2015; Mendola et al., 2015; Naimi et al., 2016; Nguyen et al., 2016; Pearce et al., 2016; Zhang et al., 2015) of the counterfactual-based approach.

A Note on how We will View the Path Analysis Approach in this Chapter
The path analysis and 'causal inference' approaches to mediation analysis are not entirely different, and should not in general be viewed as being in opposition to each other. Most notably, Judea Pearl, one of the founders of the modern causal inference school, wrote one of the first and seminal papers on causal mediation analysis; he explicitly uses SEMs as the cornerstone of his approach and thus firmly regards the path analysis approach as a subset of the causal inference approach, rather than in competition with it Bollen and Pearl (2013). However, other advocates and users of SEMs, and specifically the approach to mediation analysis contained within it, take a less formally causal view of the approach; at the other extreme from Pearl, SEMs are (mis-)used purely as a set of statistical regression models, and it is this interpretation which has most often been presumed by mediation analysis practitioners. Indeed, the approach is often called *statistical mediation analysis* MacKinnon (2008) in order to contrast it with the counterfactual-based approach often labelled *causal mediation analysis*. A comparison between Pearl's view of the path analysis approach and the causal inference approach would be vacuous, since they are essentially one and the same; for this reason, together with the reason that Pearl's view is not in our experience the one most commonly adopted in practice, we will take a purely statistical interpretation of the path analysis approach when describing it below. We do so with a knowing caveat that this is unrepresentative of the position taken by some proponents and users of the approach (Bollen & Pearl, 2013; Chen & Pearl, 2013).

In the next sections we describe and compare the above two approaches in a setting with only one mediator of interest and where the outcome is either continuous or binary; we discuss the important issue of intermediate confounding. In Sect. 1.3 we review extensions to time-to-event outcomes, and in Sect. 1.4 we apply the methods discussed to an example dataset.

1.2 Alternative Approaches

Consider the simplified setting shown in Fig. 1.2 which includes only one mediator. We denote the exposure by X, the mediator by M, and the outcome by Y. In addition we include in the diagram a $(p \times 1)$ column vector $\mathbf{C} = (C_1, C_2, \ldots, C_p)^T$ representing a set of p potential confounders of the X–Y, X–M and M–Y relationships.[1]

[1]Note that T represents matrix transposition, so that $\mathbf{C}$ is $(p \times 1)$ even though $(C_1, C_2, \ldots, C_p)$ is a $(1 \times p)$ row vector. This will be useful for writing regression equations later. Also note that, for now, an informal notion of "confounding" is adopted, but see Sect. 1.2.2.3 for the formal definition.

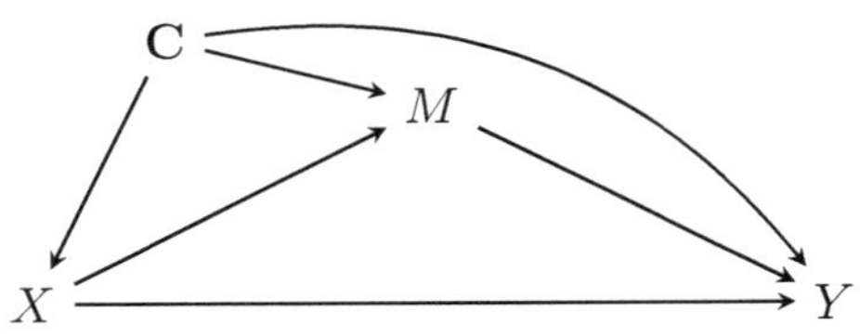

Fig. 1.2 Simplified diagram where X represents the exposure, M the mediator, and Y the outcome. The figure also includes $\mathbf{C}$ a set of potential confounders of the X–Y, X–M and M–Y relationships

To focus only on issues relating to mediation, we presume that the data on these variables are complete and unaffected by measurement error.

1.2.1 The Path Analysis Approach

Almost exclusively using linear regression models, the mediation analysis literature linked to path analysis follows one of two different, but equivalent, procedures, known as the methods of *difference* or *multiplication* of coefficients Baron and Kenny (1986).

Supposing Y and M both to be continuous variables, a linear regression model for Y given the exposure X, the mediator M and confounders $\mathbf{C}$ is specified as:

$$E(Y|X = x, M = m, \mathbf{C} = \mathbf{c}) = \beta_0 + \beta_x x + \beta_m m + \boldsymbol{\beta}_c^T \mathbf{c}, \tag{1.1}$$

where $E(Y|X = x, M = m, \mathbf{C} = \mathbf{c})$ is the expectation (or mean) of Y in the subset of the population of interest for whom $X = x$, $M = m$ and $\mathbf{C} = \mathbf{c}$. $\boldsymbol{\beta}_c$ denotes a $(p \times 1)$ column vector of p parameters, the jth of which is β_{cj}, so that $\boldsymbol{\beta}_c^T \mathbf{c} = \beta_{c1} c_1 + \beta_{c2} c_2 + \cdots + \beta_{cp} c_p$. Since M is included in the model, the parameter β_x intuitively does not include the effect mediated by M, and thus it is interpreted as the direct effect of X on Y not mediated by M.

In the *method of difference*, to estimate the indirect effect, another linear regression model for Y given the exposure X and confounders $\mathbf{C}$ (but not M) is specified:

$$E(Y|X = x, \mathbf{C} = \mathbf{c}) = \gamma_0 + \gamma_x x + \boldsymbol{\gamma}_c^T \mathbf{c}. \tag{1.2}$$

Since M is now not included in the model, the effect of X through M is included in the parameter γ_x and thus this is interpreted as the *total effect* of X on Y.

The difference between the total and the direct effect,

$$\gamma_x - \beta_x,$$

is then interpreted as the *indirect effect*, the effect mediated by M. Even when this difference is not formally calculated, a similar logic is often employed: a model for Y given X and $\mathbf{C}$ is fitted twice, once without and once with the mediator included in the model. The extent to which the coefficient of X changes is deemed to be indicative of the extent to which the effect is mediated by M.

In the *method of multiplication*, to estimate the indirect effect, a linear regression model for M given X and $\mathbf{C}$ is specified,

$$E\left(M \mid X = x, \mathbf{C} = \mathbf{c}\right) = \alpha_0 + \alpha_x x + \boldsymbol{\alpha}_c^T \mathbf{c}. \tag{1.3}$$

Using the *path tracing rule* of path analysis (Bollen, 1989; Wright, 1934), the coefficients along the path from X to Y that involve M (i.e. in this case, $X \to M \to Y$) are multiplied, so that the indirect effect is $\alpha_x \beta_m$. Intuitively, this makes sense by considering that a unit change in X would lead to a α_x change in M, and hence, in turn, a $\alpha_x \beta_m$ change in Y via M.

It can easily be shown that, in the setting described above:

$$\gamma_x - \beta_x = \alpha_x \beta_m$$

and therefore that the difference and multiplication methods (for simple linear models) are equivalent.

In both, estimation of the models' parameters is carried out by ordinary least square (OLS) (equivalently, maximum likelihood) and combined to obtain estimators of the indirect effect. Standard errors for the estimated indirect effects—$(\hat{\gamma}_x - \hat{\beta}_x)$ or $\hat{\alpha}_x \hat{\beta}_m$—are estimated either via the delta method or bootstrapping MacKinnon, Lockwood, Hoffman, West, & Sheets, (2002), with the former requiring additional assumptions (such as homoscedasticity of errors) depending on the precise formulae used.

Note that models (1.1)–(1.3) are often written with Y and M on the left-hand sides, instead of $E(Y|\cdot)$ and $E(M|\cdot)$, and additive error terms are included on the right-hand sides. The precise meaning of such error terms depends on the view (statistical or causal) taken of the model, and confusion often follows. See (Bollen & Pearl, 2013; Chen & Pearl, 2013) for a full discussion of this point. By writing the models as we have written them above, we make explicit that they are simply statistical models, in line with the caveat we gave in the second half of the Introduction.

1.2.1.1 Extensions and Criticisms

The difference method, since it does not rely on a model for M, can be used also when the relationship between M and $(X, \mathbf{C})$ cannot be described using the linear regression model (1.3), e.g. when M is binary, or when there is effect modification by some of the confounders of the effect of X on M. Also, since it makes no use of the coefficient β_m, it can also be used when there is effect modification by $\mathbf{C}$ of the effect of M on Y. The product method, on the other hand, extends to deal with any number of path-specific effects through any number of mediators, as long as all relationships can be described using simple linear regression models as above. Beyond this, however, these simple approaches are difficult to generalise, e.g. to settings with non-linearities, as has been pointed out (e.g. VanderWeele, 2009; VanderWeele and Vansteelandt, 2015), and as reviewed below.

Reliance on linearity Without more formal work (as has been done in the literature on causal mediation analysis; see Sect. 1.2.2) it is unclear how the difference or the product method would generalise if the model for Y included an X–M interaction as in

$$E(Y|X = x, M = m, \mathbf{C} = \mathbf{c}) = \beta_0 + \beta_x x + \beta_m m + \beta_{xm} xm + \boldsymbol{\beta}_c^T \mathbf{c},$$

or if the model included other non-linearities in X and/or (for the product method) M, such as

$$E(Y|X = x, M = m, \mathbf{C} = \mathbf{c}) = \beta_0 + \beta_x x + \beta_{x2} x^2 + \beta_{xc_j} x c_j + \beta_m m + \beta_{m2} m^2 + \boldsymbol{\beta}_c^T \mathbf{c}.$$

With more than one term in x on the right-hand sides of these equations, it seems intuitively obvious that β_x no longer captures the direct effect; so what does? Without a model-free definition of what we mean by *direct effect* (see criticism "Lack of causal formalism"), it is difficult to know how to proceed.

Furthermore if Y were a binary or time-to-event outcome modelled by logistic or Cox regression, even in the absence of an X–M interaction or other non-linearities in the linear predictor, the use of the path tracing rule, and hence the product method, would no longer be justified. The difference method, on the other hand, would run into problems of model incompatibility and non-collapsibility: if, for example, $E(Y|\mathbf{C}, X, M)$ is a logistic function of $(\mathbf{C}, X, M)$, then it is not in general a logistic function of $(\mathbf{C}, X)$, and the comparison of the two conditional odds ratios for the effect of X in the two models would not be comparable since one would be additionally conditional on M, rendering them different even in the absence of any effect of X on M. However, since non-collapsibility moves effects away from the null, it has been argued Jiang and VanderWeele (2015) that the difference method in such settings is conservative for assessing mediation when both the direct and indirect effects are in the same direction.

Non-linearities involving only the confounders can easily be included in these models, and some exploration in the causal inference liteature of the validity of these simple approaches in the presence of non-linearities beyond those involving only confounders has uncovered a few special cases where they can still be applied (Jiang & VanderWeele, 2015; VanderWeele & Vansteelandt, 2010), but in general their use is restricted to simple linear regression models as described above, with most extensions away from full linearity (see, for example, Hayes & Preacher, 2010; Winship & Mare, 1982) shown to be at best approximate.

***M*–*Y* confounding** The models from which the direct and indirect effects were derived include the variables $\mathbf{C}$. If this vector were insufficient to control for the confounding of the relationships between X, M and Y, the parameters and combinations

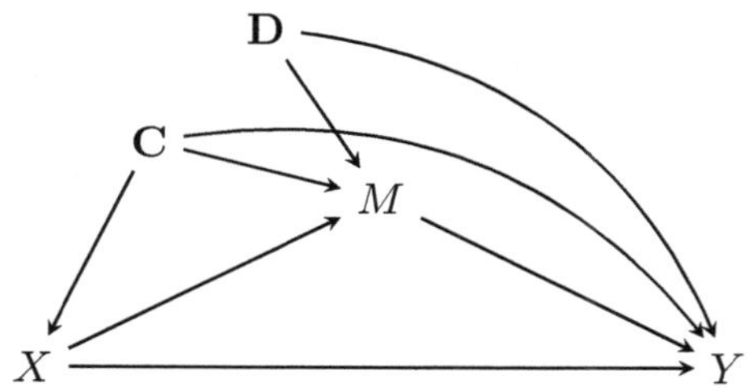

Fig. 1.3 M–Y confounding

of parameters defined above would not capture the desired direct and indirect effects, even if the strong linearity constraints were satisfied.

Although the need to control for confounders is broadly recognised, it has often not been sufficiently stressed that this includes potential confounders of M and Y, such that confounding is an important concern in mediation analysis, even in studies in which the exposure X is randomised Emsley, Dunn, & White (2010).

To see this let $\mathbf{D}$ denote such confounders (Fig. 1.3). Including X, M and $\mathbf{C}$ but not $\mathbf{D}$ in model (1.1) would open up a non-causal path from X to Y via M and $\mathbf{D}$ because M is a collider along this path, and conditioning on a collider (as done in (1.1)) creates an association between the variables that influence it, in this case X and $\mathbf{D}$. This is an example of *collider stratification bias* (Cole & Hernán, 2002; Greenland, 2003), and it means that the coefficient β_x in model (1.1) would represent this non-causal path as well as the direct effect of interest.

Note that controlling for $\mathbf{D}$ in the model for Y, as in

$$E\left(Y\,|X = x, M = m, \mathbf{C} = \mathbf{c}, \mathbf{D} = \mathbf{d}\right) = \beta_0^{\dagger} + \beta_x^{\dagger} x + \beta_m^{\dagger} m + \boldsymbol{\beta}_c^{\dagger T} \mathbf{c} + \beta_d^{\dagger T} \mathbf{d}$$

would render the path blocked again, so that $\beta_x^{\dagger}$ would represent the direct effect we are after, provided again that the linear regression model, now including $\mathbf{D}$ too, is correctly specified.

Exposure-induced confounding Complications arise however if any of the M–Y confounders is influenced by X. As is common in the literature, we denote such M–Y confounders affected by X by $\mathbf{L}$ (Fig. 1.4). This type of confounding is also labelled *intermediate* to contrast it with *background* confounding (such as that represented by $\mathbf{C}$ or $\mathbf{D}$) VanderWeele, Vansteelandt, and Robins (2014). As discussed in the previous paragraph, common causes of M and Y should be controlled for to avoid inducing collider bias into the estimation of the direct effect. However, if such confounders are intermediate, like $\mathbf{L}$, this would also block part of the direct effect from X to Y, since $\mathbf{L}$ contributes to the path $X \to \mathbf{L} \to Y$ that originates from X but does not involve M.

By extending the model to include a equations for $\mathbf{L}$, we could attempt to address this problem using the path tracing rules. Consider this set of linear regression models, for a (univariate) continuous L, together with M and Y:

Fig. 1.4 Exposure induced confounding of the M–Y relationship

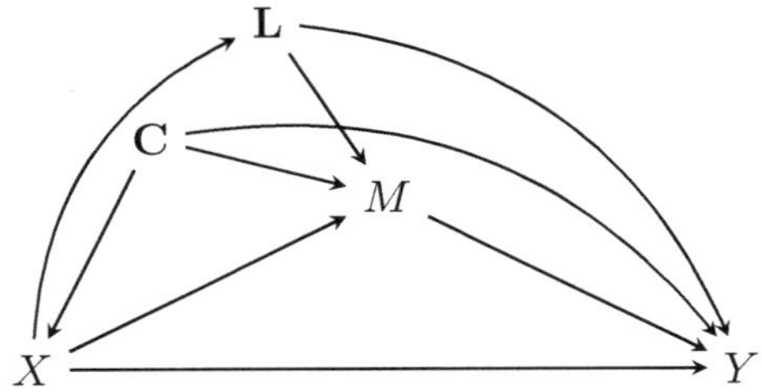

$$
\begin{aligned}
E\left(L\,|X=x,\mathbf{C}=\mathbf{c}\right) &= \delta_0^* + \delta_x^* x + \boldsymbol{\delta}_c^{*T}\mathbf{c} \\
E\left(M\,|X=x,L=l,\mathbf{C}=\mathbf{c}\right) &= \alpha_0^* + \alpha_x^* x + \alpha_l^* l + \boldsymbol{\alpha}_c^{*T}\mathbf{c} \\
E\left(Y\,|X=x,L=l,M=m,\mathbf{C}=\mathbf{c}\right) &= \beta_0^* + \beta_x^* x + \beta_l^* l + \beta_m^* m + \boldsymbol{\beta}_c^{*T}\mathbf{c}
\end{aligned}
$$

Using Wright's path-tracing rule on this extended model we find that the effect mediated by M is $(\alpha_x^*\beta_m^* + \delta_x^*\alpha_l^*\beta_m^*)$ and the effect not mediated by M is $(\beta_x^* + \delta_x^*\beta_l^*)$. This offers a sensible solution to the problem of intermediate confounding, provided there is no further confounding of L and Y. If there were, then what if that further confounding were also intermediate? It would seem that we would need to go on and on adding more and more equations, relying on more and more linearity assumptions. In fact, this is not fully the case De Stavola, Daniel, Ploubidis, and Micali (2015), but uncovering slight relaxations of the apparent SEM assumptions is only feasible when adopting the more formal approach of Sect. 1.2.2.

Lack of causal formalism The formal view taken above is that the parameters of interest, such as β_x, are simply parameters in a statistical model. Our intuitive and informal discussion accompanying this, however, has been heightened with some loose causal interpretation. Since this causal interpretation is left to our intuition, and since intuition can only take us so far, we have hit the stumbling blocks outlined in "Reliance on linearity"–"Exposure-induced confounding" above. A more general criticism of the approach we have thus far described is therefore that it is not clear what exactly a *direct effect* and an *indirect effect* mean, and thus the assumptions under which they can be identified from data are also left somewhat vague. Moreover, although the linking of β_x and $\alpha_x\beta_m$ with direct and indirect effects, respectively, seems reasonable in the linear setting for which they are described, it is apparent that more formal notions are needed if correct generalisations are to be made, even to settings that deviate only slightly from those above.

Mediation enquiries are causal enquiries. The very notion that M is *intermediate* between X and Y is meaningless if only associations are being considered, since associations are inherently symmetric and hence without order. It is perhaps not surprising therefore that mediation enquiries have lent themselves to a more formal treatment within the counterfactual-based causal inference literature, spurred on most recently by numerous contributions by VanderWeele and co-authors Valeri and VanderWeele (2009), VanderWeele (2010, 2014), VanderWeele and Shpitser 2009a,

VanderWeele and Vansteelandt (2010, 2012), VanderWeele et al. (2012), Vansteelandt (2012), Vansteelandt and VanderWeele (2013).

1.2.2 *The Counterfactual-Based Approach*

In order to define precisely what is meant by a causal effect, the causal inference literature has adopted various additions to standard statistical notation, the most popular of which has been counterfactuals or potential outcomes Robins (1986), Rubin (1974). These encapsulate intuitive notions of causation such as "how different would Y have been had X been different?". Mediation effects have been formally defined in terms of such hypothetical quantities and their extensions Robins and Greenland (1992), as we describe below. Note, however, that identical or similar definitions, respectively, have been proposed using alternative causal notations (Geneletti, 2007; Pearl, 2001).

The main advantage of adopting a rigorous and explicitly causal approach is that it formalises and generalises the definitions of direct and indirect effects so that they no longer depend on the specification of a particular statistical model. The definitions therefore extend to any type of outcome and mediator, without restricting the relationships to be linear. The unambiguous nature of these formal definitions of mediation estimands (i.e. the quantities of interest whose true values are to be estimated) together with the fact that they are divorced from the statistical models we may use to estimate them, have allowed the elucidation of the assumptions under which they can be identified from the data at hand, together with an array of possible estimation methods for doing so.

In this section we give a brief overview of the most commonly used counterfactual-based mediation estimands, and of the main assumptions necessary to identify them; however see the recently published book by VanderWeele (2015) both for more breadth and depth on all the aspects discussed.

1.2.2.1 Definitions

The following counterfactuals are used in the definitions of mediation effects.

- Let $Y(x)$ and $M(x)$ be the potential values of, respectively, the outcome and the mediator, that would have occurred had the exposure been set to the value x, where x may be different from the actual value that the exposure was observed to take, X;
- Let $Y(x, m)$ be the potential value of Y had X been set to x and M to m;
- Let $Y(x, M(x^*))$ be the potential value of Y, also called a *nested counterfactual*, that would have occurred had X been set to x and M to $M(x^*)$.

The total causal effect (TCE) of X on Y, expressed as a difference in population mean potential outcomes, comparing levels x and x^* of X is:

$$\text{TCE}(x, x^*) = E\{Y(x^*)\} - E\{Y(x)\},$$

i.e. it is the difference between the mean outcome that would hypothetically be observed if everyone in the population were to receive exposure level x^* versus if everyone were to receive exposure level x. For example, for a binary X, x and x^* would be 0 and 1, respectively, and the TCE would be defined as:

$$\text{TCE} = E\{Y(1)\} - E\{Y(0)\}.$$

In the following, we briefly review similar contrasts that capture instead various types of direct and indirect effects. For simplicity, in each case we express them, as above, as differences in population mean potential outcomes (equivalent to risk differences for binary outcomes) although other contrasts, such as risk ratios, odds ratios, as well as effects conditional on baseline variables, can be used, as given in the Web Appendix that accompanies this chapter. Also for simplicity, we give these definitions for a binary X, so that x and x^* take values 0 and 1.

The controlled direct effect The *controlled direct effect* of X on Y when M is controlled at m (CDE(m)) (Pearl, 2001; Robins and Greenland, 1992) is defined as:

$$\text{CDE}(m) = E\left\{Y\left(1, m\right)\right\} - E\left\{Y\left(0, m\right)\right\}.$$

The CDE(m) is a comparison of two hypothetical scenarios where in the first X is set to 1, and in the second to 0, while in both M is set to m. Since M is set to take the same value in the two scenarios, CDE(m) captures a (type of) direct effect of X on Y not mediated through M. Note that this definition requires imagining that the mediator be set at a fixed value uniformly across the population.

For example, if (binary) childhood disadvantage (1 = disadvantaged, 0 = not disadvantaged) were the exposure, level of education received the mediator, and adult BMI the outcome, then the controlled direct effect at level "high school" of the mediator would be the difference in mean adult BMI in the population of interest comparing two hypothetical situations, one in which everyone were disadvantaged in childhood, and the other in which noone were disadvantaged, but in both situations everyone would hypothetically have finished high school, with noone going beyond high school.

Unfortunately, there is no indirect counterpart to the controlled direct effect. Were we to attempt to define a controlled indirect effect as the difference between the total causal effect of X on Y and the controlled direct effect above, the resulting quantity would not in general possess the basic properties that we would expect of a sensible definition of an indirect effect. For example, such a quantity would in general be non-zero even in the absence of an effect of X on M VanderWeele (2009b). For this, and other reasons, alternative counterfactual mediation effects have been defined.

Natural direct and indirect effects The *natural direct effect* (NDE) of X on Y (Pearl, 2001; Robins & Greenland, 1992) is defined as:

$$\mathrm{NDE} = E\{Y(1, M(0))\} - E\{Y(0, M(0))\}.$$

The NDE is also a comparison of two hypothetical scenarios where X is set to 0 versus 1, but M is set to take the value $M(0)$ in both scenarios. This is a so-called natural value because it is specific to each individual were that individual's exposure set at 0. Again, since for a given individual M is set at the same value ($M(0)$) in the two scenarios, NDE captures a (type of) direct effect of X on Y.

Going back to our example, the NDE above is the difference in mean adult BMI in the population were everyone versus noone to be disadvantaged, but with each individual's education level set to what it would have been had he or she not been disadvantaged. It therefore allows each individual to have a different education level, but such that this education level is not affected (for the purposes of this contrast) by disadvantage. It therefore asks the question, "what would the effect of disadvantage be on BMI if it had no effect on education?".

The *natural indirect effect* (NIE) (Robins, 1992; Robins and Greenland, 2003) is defined as:

$$\mathrm{NIE} = E\{Y(1, M(1))\} - E\{Y(1, M(0))\}.$$

This is a comparison of two hypothetical scenarios, where X is set to 1 in both, while M changes from its value had X been set to 1 to its value had X been set to 0. This captures the part of the effect of X on Y transmitted by M.

In our example, it is the difference in mean adult BMI in the population were everyone to be disadvantaged, but comparing a situation in which each individual's education level would be what it would have been had he or she been disadvantaged versus what it would have been had he or she not been disadvantaged. It therefore isolates the part of the effect of disadvantage on BMI that is transmitted through education level.

The NDE and NIE have the property that their sum is the total causal effect, TCE,

$$\begin{aligned}\mathrm{NDE} + \mathrm{NIE} &= E\{Y(1, M(0))\} - E\{Y(0, M(0))\} \\ &\quad + E\{Y(1, M(1))\} - E\{Y(1, M(0))\} \\ &= E\{Y(1)\} - E\{Y(0)\} \\ &= \mathrm{TCE}.\end{aligned}$$

In other words the TCE decomposes into the sum of the natural direct and natural indirect effects.[2] This decomposition applies in general, i.e. it does not depend on

[2]One important subtlety that we do not consider further in this chapter is that an alternative partitioning of the total effect in terms of alternative definitions of natural effects is given by $\mathrm{TCE} = E\{Y(1, M(1))\} - E\{Y(0, M(1))\} + E\{Y(0, M(1))\} - E\{Y(0, M(0))\}$. In other words, the definitions of NDE and NIE given above are not unique. Indeed, reversing the coding of X leads in general to direct and indirect effects of different magnitudes (not just different signs), which is somewhat unpleasing. This was acknowledged when the first definitions were given Robins and Greenland (1992), and much has been written about it since; see, for example, (Daniel, De Stavola, Cousens, & Vansteelandt, 2015; VanderWeele, 2013).

a particular model for the outcome or for the mediator, unlike the decomposition described in relation to Eqs. (1.1)–(1.3).

Interventional direct and indirect effects The randomised interventional analogues (RIA) of the NDE and NIE, are defined as (VanderWeele et al., 2014; Vansteelandt & Daniel, 2016)[3]:

$$\text{RIA-NDE} = E\left\{Y\left(1, M^*_{0|\mathbf{C}}\right)\right\} - E\left\{Y\left(0, M^*_{0|\mathbf{C}}\right)\right\} \tag{1.4}$$

$$\text{RIA-NIE} = E\left\{Y\left(1, M^*_{1|\mathbf{C}}\right)\right\} - E\left\{Y\left(1, M^*_{0|\mathbf{C}}\right)\right\} \tag{1.5}$$

where $M^*_{x|\mathbf{C}}$ is a random draw from the distribution of $M(x)$ conditional on $\mathbf{C}$. The RIA-NDE is the direct effect derived when comparing exposure versus no exposure with the mediator in both cases randomly drawn from its counterfactual distribution under no exposure (given $\mathbf{C}$), and similarly the RIA-NIE fixes the exposure at 1 but compares randomly drawing the mediator from its counterfactual distribution under exposure versus no exposure (given $\mathbf{C}$).

These are very similar to effects first introduced within the decision theory framework (Didelez, Dawid, & Geneletti, 2007; Geneletti, 2006).

Using our example, the RIA-NDE is the difference in mean adult BMI in the population were everyone versus noone to be disadvantaged, but with each individual's education level drawn from the hypothetical distribution of education level, given confounders, were everyone to be disadvantaged. The RIA-NIE is the difference in mean adult BMI in the population that would result from keeping everyone's exposure fixed at disadvantaged, and drawing each individual's education level from its hypothetical distribution were everyone to be disadvantaged versus advantaged, given confounders. Alternatively, it can be thought of as the change in mean adult BMI that would be brought about by fixing the exposure at disadvantaged for everyone, whilst shifting the conditional distribution of education level, given confounders, from what it would have been had everyone been advantaged to what it would have been had everyone been disadvantaged. The key difference between this and the natural indirect effect, is that the hypothetical shift is applied to the distribution of $M(x)$ given $\mathbf{C}$, rather than at the individual level.

These interventional effects however do not in general lead to a decomposition of the TCE. Their sum is:

$$\text{RIA-NDE} + \text{RIA-NIE} = E\left\{Y\left(1, M^*_{1|\mathbf{C}}\right)\right\} + E\left\{Y\left(0, M^*_{0|\mathbf{C}}\right)\right\}$$

and this is not in general equal to the TCE. VanderWeele et al. (2014) call $E\left\{Y\left(1, M^*_{1|\mathbf{C}}\right)\right\} + E\left\{Y\left(0, M^*_{0|\mathbf{C}}\right)\right\}$ the *overall* effect of X on Y. In any empirical

[3]Note that the definitions given here are not exactly the same as those originally given by VanderWeele et al. (2014), but rather are the closely-related definitions given by Vansteelandt and Daniel (2016).

example, both can be estimated, and thus the extent of the discrepancy assessed subject to no parametric model misspecification. Were **C** to predict $M(x)$ perfectly, then no difference would be found between the total and overall effects. The larger the influence of other variables (other than **C**) on $M(x)$, therefore, the larger we would expect the discrepancy between the total and overall effects to be.

Although the lack of exact decomposition of the TCE is a disadvantage, these interventional effects possess other desirable properties. First, they correspond to interventions that could in principle be applied, and thus are arguably more policy-relevant Vansteelandt and Daniel (2016), and second they can be identified under weaker assumptions than the corresponding natural effects, as we describe below.

1.2.2.2 Further Comparisons of the Counterfactual-Based Mediation Estimands

The controlled direct effect is sometimes said to be *prescriptive* because it imagines hypothetical scenarios in which we set both exposure and mediator to particular (known) values for everyone, something which we could in principle imagine doing, even if in practice it would be entirely unfeasible to do so; for this reason it has been argued that it is more relevant for policy makers (Naimi et al., 2014; Pearl, 2001). However, imagining that the mediator be set to exactly the same value for all is suited only to enquiries where such homogeneity would be meaningful. Examples include mediators such as infections, where it might be sensible to consider the remaining effect of the exposure were the infection hypothetically to be eradicated for all. Likewise with behaviour variables such as smoking, we might meaningfully ask about the remaining effect of the exposure if cigarette smoking were eliminated for all. However, with many of the mediators encountered in life course investigations, such as physical activity, educational achievement *etc.*, it seems far-fetched to imagine a hypothetical scenario in which everyone exercises exactly the same amount, or achieves exactly the same level of education. The fact that the CDE does not in general lead to a decomposition of the TCE into direct and indirect components is also often seen as a disadvantage, and this is particularly relevant in life course settings where multiple mediators, and hence multiple path-specific (indirect) effects are of interest (see brief discussion in Sect. 1.5).

The natural effects overcome both of the aforementioned limitations. They lead to a decomposition of the TCE, and do not require that we imagine scenarios in which the mediator is the same for everyone. In the case of an infection, for example, the natural direct effect would capture the remaining effect of the exposure on the outcome, were its effect on infection to be eliminated, so that infection status for each individual would remain at what it would have been had the individual been unexposed; those who would have had the infection for reasons other than the exposure, would still have the infection in the imagined comparative scenarios. In this sense the natural effects capture effects that are closer to reality, and have for this reason been labelled more *descriptive* (Naimi et al., 2014; Pearl, 2001). A disadvantage is that we could not learn, even in an experimental setting, about the joint distribution of the potential value of the mediator in the absence of the exposure and the potential value for the outcome in the presence of the exposure, and—for reasons that are apparent just by looking at the so-called *nested* counterfactual $Y(1, M(0))$ involved in the definitions—it turns out that knowledge of this joint distribution (conditional on confounders) is required for the natural effects to be identified. The reason for this difficulty in identification is directly related to our discussion of the first (desirable) property of the controlled direct effect: it corresponds to an intervention that in principle we could do; this cannot be said of the natural effects, not even in principle, since they require knowledge of how $M(0)$ and $Y(1, m)$ are linked at an individual level.

The interventional analogue effects do away with the need for knowledge of this individual link, by imagining not that M be set to $M(0)$ but to a draw from its distribution given $\mathbf{C}$, and thus they can be identified under less Herculian assumptions. The price to pay is then that the effects do not lead to a decomposition of the total causal effect, but rather a similar, but not identical, overall effect.

As so often in statistics, and in causal inference in particular, there is a trade-off between how closely an estimand corresponds to what we truly wish to learn about, and the strength of the assumptions needed to identify it. We now turn to a more thorough examination of these assumptions.

1.2.2.3 Assumptions

The advantage of the definitions we have reviewed above is that, by appealing to counterfactuals, they more precisely and explicitly capture the notions of direct and indirect effects than do the statistical parameters of the previous section. An apparent corresponding *dis*advantage, however, is that it is not immediately clear how we can learn about these effects from data which inevitably do not contain within them the counterfactual variables involved in the definitions. Assumptions are needed therefore to connect aspects of the distribution of the observed data to the defined causal estimands; this process is known as identification.

Due to this step, which involves the many assumptions listed below, it may seem that the counterfactual-based approach relies on more assumptions; this is strictly speaking true, if, when using the path analysis approach, we would give our parameters of interest only their statistical interpretation, e.g. that

$$\beta_x = E(Y|X = x + 1, M = m, \mathbf{C} = \mathbf{c}) - E(Y|X = x, M = m, \mathbf{C} = \mathbf{c}).$$

However, as soon as we interpret the above as a *direct effect* of X on Y unmediated by M, then—implicitly—we are relying on additional assumptions in order to justify this heightened interpretation. By clearly defining direct and indirect effects using counterfactuals, these additional assumptions can be made explicit.

Stronger assumptions are needed to identify the natural effects than the controlled direct effect, with those sufficient to identify the interventional effects lying between the two. The technical assumptions of *no interference* and *consistency* are needed, as well as no unmeasured confounding assumptions, also known as *conditional exchangeability* assumptions.[4] The identification of natural effects relies on an additional assumption, namely the *cross-world independence* assumption, or a slightly weaker alternative. We now discuss each of these assumption types in turn, before noting which assumptions are sufficient for identifying the various mediation effects introduced in this section.

No interference By writing $Y(x, m)$ to mean the value that Y would take for an individual if X for that individual had been set to x and M for that individual to m, we are already assuming that what the exposure and mediator variables of *other* individuals may have been set to would not have an impact on the outcome for the individual in question. This assumption is known as *no interference* (for the outcome) (Cox, 1958; Hudgens & Halloran, 2008; Rubin, 1980; Tchetgen & VanderWeele, 2012). This is typically assumed when identifying all of the mediation estimands above. In addition, for the natural effects, no interference for the mediator is also typically assumed, namely that the exposure for one individual does not influence the mediator of another. If sufficient data on the structure of interference patterns are available, e.g. in some studies of social networks, then progress can be made by modelling interference when it is present (Tchetgen Tchetgen, & VanderWeele, 2012; VanderWeele, 2009c), but we don't consider these extensions further in this chapter.

Consistency *Consistency* (for the outcome) states that, for each x and m, the potential outcome $Y(x, m)$ is equal to the observed outcome Y among subjects with observed exposure $X = x$ and observed mediator $M = m$ (Cole & Frangakis, 2009; Hernán & Taubman, 2008; Pearl, 2010; VanderWeele, 2009c). Similarly, consistency for the mediator states that the potential mediator value $M(x)$ is equal to the observed mediator M among subjects with observed exposure $X = x$. In short, consistency ensures that when interpreting causal effect estimates as a comparison of what would have been seen under particular hypothetical interventions, the interventions we imagine are not further removed from the data than is justified Daniel, De Stavola, & Vansteelandt, (inpress).

Conditional exchangeability The concept of 'no unmeasured confounding' has been formalised in the causal inference literature in the form of conditional exchangeability assumptions Greenland and Robins (1986). For mediation estimands, the relevant versions of conditional exchangeability are the following VanderWeele and Vansteelandt (2009):

CE (i): When M is set to m, the remaining effect of the exposure X on the outcome Y is unconfounded, conditional on $\mathbf{C}$; mathematically, this is written as

$$Y(x, m) \perp\!\!\!\perp X \,|\mathbf{C} = \mathbf{c}\ ,\ \ \forall x, \mathbf{c},$$

[4]This is since we are using approaches that deal with confounding by adjustment/weighting etc, rather than approaches that rely on having measured instrumental variables Burgess (2015).

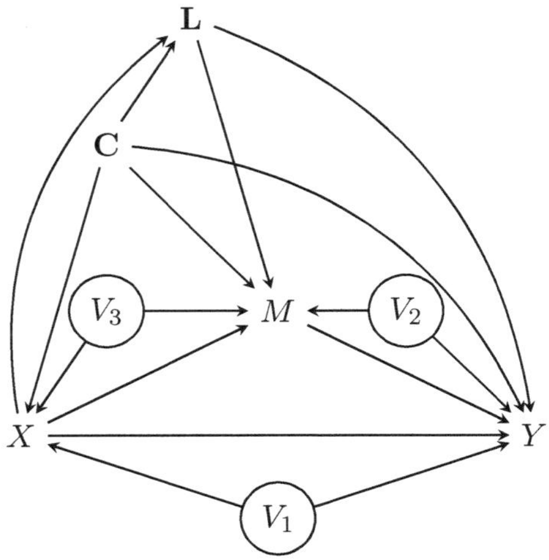

Fig. 1.5 Identification assumptions: conditional exchangeability

where $A \perp\!\!\!\perp B|C$ stands for "A is conditionally independent of B given C" and $\forall$ means "for all".
Graphically, it is the assumption that there can be no unmeasured common causes V_1 of X and Y in Fig. 1.5.[5]
CE (ii): The effect of the mediator M on the outcome Y is unconfounded, conditional on X and $\mathbf{C}$ (and intermediate confounder(s) $\mathbf{L} = (L_1, L_2, \ldots, L_q)^T$ if applicable); mathematically,

$$Y(x, m) \perp\!\!\!\perp M \,|\mathbf{C} = \mathbf{c}, X = x, \mathbf{L} = \mathbf{l}\ ,\ \forall x, m, \mathbf{c}, \mathbf{l}.$$

This corresponds to no unmeasured common causes V_2 of M and Y in Fig. 1.5.
CE (iii): The effect of the exposure X on the mediator M is unconfounded, conditional on $\mathbf{C}$; mathematically

$$M(x) \perp\!\!\!\perp X \,|\mathbf{C} = \mathbf{c}\ ,\ \forall x, \mathbf{c}.$$

This corresponds to no unmeasured common causes V_3 of X and M in Fig. 1.5.

Note that unmeasured common causes of $\mathbf{L}$ and Y could be added to Fig. 1.5 without violating any of the assumptions above.

For the CDE(m) sufficient assumptions for identification are: no interference for the outcome, consistency for the outcome, CE (i) and CE (ii). For the interventional effects sufficient assumptions for identification are: no interference for the outcome and the mediator, consistency for the outcome and the mediator, CE (i), CE (ii), and

[5]Note that the mathematical representation of this assumption makes it clear that in fact unmeasured common causes of X and M (i.e. V_3 in Fig. 1.5), which would constitute a form of unmeasured confounding of X and Y, is not prohibited by this assumption.

CE (iii). However, even this latter set of assumptions is not sufficient to identify the natural effects.

Cross-world independence Natural direct and indirect effects are identified if, in addition to no interference (for outcome and mediator), consistency (for outcome and mediator) and CE (i)–(iii), the following, so called *cross-world* independence (CWI) assumption holds:

$$Y(1, m) \perp\!\!\!\perp M(0) \,|\mathbf{C} = \mathbf{c} \;, \;\; \forall m, \mathbf{c}.$$

Pearl (2001) and many others (most notably Richardson & Robins, 2013; Robins & Richardson, 2010) have discussed the CWI assumption and its consequences. It is a difficult assumption to understand because $Y(1, m)$ and $M(0)$ could never be observed on the same individual even in a hypothetical experiment; hence the conditional independence we must contemplate is *across two different worlds*. Moreover, one serious consequence of this assumption is that it rules out the presence of exposure-induced confounders $\mathbf{L}$ of the M–Y relationship. With the usual long time gap between the exposure and the mediators involved in life course epidemiology, intermediate confounders are very plausible and hence the CWI assumption unrealistic.

Some slightly weaker and/or alternative assumptions to CWI have been proposed in the literature to achieve identification of natural effects in the presence of intermediate confounding (Petersen, Sinisi, & van der Laan, 2006; Robins & Greenland, 1992; Tchetgen Tchetgen & VanderWeele, 2014), but these impose parametric and/or 'no interaction' restrictions which are also very strong and, with the exception of one proposal by Tchetgen Tchetgen Tchetgen Tchetgen and VanderWeele (2014), untestable.

In contrast, the identifying assumptions for the interventional effects do not involve either the CWI nor the aforementioned alternatives, and therefore make them an attractive option for life course investigations.

1.2.2.4 Identification

In this section, we revisit the steps given elsewhere (Pearl, 2001; VanderWeele, 2015; VanderWeele & Vansteelandt, 2009) that show how the assumptions above lead to the identification of the counterfactual-based mediation estimands, i.e. how, under the assumptions above, the mediation estimands can be re-written in terms of aspects of the distribution of the observed data. It is useful to follow these steps in order to appreciate how and when the various assumptions are used in the identification of the different estimands. The steps that follow also give further insights into the difference between the estimands, as well as highlighting how the counterfactual-based approach to mediation analysis overcomes some of the limitations of the more traditional approaches. However, those with a lower tolerance for mathematical detail may wish to take this section on trust and proceed to Sect. 1.2.2.5.

Identification of the controlled direct effect We start with the controlled direct effect,

$$\text{CDE}(m) = E\left\{Y(1,m) - Y(0,m)\right\}.$$

First note that identifying $E\left\{Y(x,m)\right\}$ is sufficient to identify CDE(m), by first substituting $x = 1$ and then $x = 0$ and finding the difference between the two expressions. We focus therefore on $E\left\{Y(x,m)\right\}$. First, we rewrite it, using the law of total expectation (which says that, for discrete B, $E(A) = \sum_b E(A|B = b)\text{Pr}(B = b)$), as:

$$E\left\{Y(x,m)\right\} = \sum_{\mathbf{c}} E\left\{Y(x,m)|\,\mathbf{C} = \mathbf{c}\right\} \text{Pr}\left(\mathbf{C} = \mathbf{c}\right). \tag{1.6}$$

Note that in the above we are supposing that all the variables in **C** are discrete. Were they to be continuous, we would replace the probability by a density function, and the summation sign by an integral, and for mixtures of continuous and discrete variables we could use dominating measures. The principles are exactly the same, however, as in the all discrete case, and so for simplicity of notation, we use summations and probabilities.

Assumption CE (i) gives us the license to condition on $X = x$ in the expectation on the right-hand side of (1.6), to give the following:

$$E\left\{Y(x,m)\right\} = \sum_{\mathbf{c}} E\left\{Y(x,m)|\,\mathbf{C} = \mathbf{c}, X = x\right\} \text{Pr}\left(\mathbf{C} = \mathbf{c}\right). \tag{1.7}$$

This is since CE (i) asserts that $Y(x,m)$ is conditionally independent of X given **C**. Thus, we are not changing the conditional expectation above by additionally conditioning on $X = x$.

Further use of the law of total expectation then lets us re-write the RHS of (1.7) to obtain the following:

$$E\left\{Y(x,m)\right\} = \sum_{\mathbf{c},\mathbf{l}} E\left\{Y(x,m)|\,\mathbf{C} = \mathbf{c}, X = x, \mathbf{L} = \mathbf{l}\right\}$$
$$\text{Pr}\left(\mathbf{L} = \mathbf{l}\,|X = x, \mathbf{C} = \mathbf{c}\right) \text{Pr}\left(\mathbf{C} = \mathbf{c}\right) \tag{1.8}$$

where again we suppose that **L** contains only discrete variables, but continuous variables could easily be accommodated as explained above.[6]

Assumption CE (ii) then gives us the license to condition on $M = m$ in the conditional expectation on the RHS of (1.2.2.4), to obtain:

[6]Note that although it may appear more complicated, we are only using the identity $E(A) = \sum_b E(A|B = b)\text{Pr}(B = b)$, except now that we condition on X and **C** throughout. In other words, we are using $E(A|C) = \sum_b E(A|B = b, C)\text{Pr}(B = b|C)$ with $C = \{X, \mathbf{C}\}$, $A = Y(x,m)$ and $B = \mathbf{L}$.

$$E\{Y(x,m)\} = \sum_{\mathbf{c},\mathbf{l}} E\{Y(x,m)|\,\mathbf{C}=\mathbf{c}, X=x, \mathbf{L}=\mathbf{l}, M=m\}$$
$$\Pr(\mathbf{L}=\mathbf{l}\,|X=x, \mathbf{C}=\mathbf{c})\Pr(\mathbf{C}=\mathbf{c})$$

since CE (ii) asserts that $Y(x, m)$ is conditionally independent of M given $\mathbf{C}$ and $\mathbf{L}$ when $X = x$.

Finally, by the assumption of consistency for the outcome, we can replace $Y(x, m)$ by Y in the conditional expectation above to obtain:

$$E\{Y(x,m)\} = \sum_{\mathbf{c},\mathbf{l}} E(Y|\,\mathbf{C}=\mathbf{c}, X=x, \mathbf{L}=\mathbf{l}, M=m)$$
$$\Pr(\mathbf{L}=\mathbf{l}\,|X=x, \mathbf{C}=\mathbf{c})\Pr(\mathbf{C}=\mathbf{c}).$$

This implies, upon substituting $x = 1$ and $x = 0$ into the above and taking the difference between the two, that:

$$\text{CDE}(m) = \sum_{\mathbf{c},\mathbf{l}} E(Y|\,\mathbf{C}=\mathbf{c}, X=1, \mathbf{L}=\mathbf{l}, M=m)\Pr(\mathbf{L}=\mathbf{l}\,|X=1, \mathbf{C}=\mathbf{c})\Pr(\mathbf{C}=\mathbf{c})$$
$$-\sum_{\mathbf{c},\mathbf{l}} E(Y|\,\mathbf{C}=\mathbf{c}, X=0, \mathbf{L}=\mathbf{l}, M=m)\Pr(\mathbf{L}=\mathbf{l}\,|X=0, \mathbf{C}=\mathbf{c})\Pr(\mathbf{C}=\mathbf{c}). \tag{1.9}$$

The identification steps above fulfill a very important role: they have led to equating the causal estimand CDE(m), the mean difference between two unobservable counterfactuals, to an expression that involves only aspects of the distribution of the observed data. This does not mean that our work is done, since these aspects (conditional expectations, probabilities etc) are typically unknown and require estimation using a sample of data. But at least this task (of learning about unknown features of the joint distribution of the observed data) is what traditional statistical tools are designed to accomplish. The seemingly abstract and intractable task of learning about aspects of the distribution of unobservable quantities, has, under a set of clear assumptions, been made much more tractable through identification.

Comparison of the CDE with β_x Eq. (1.9) above applies irrespective of the nature of the mediator and the outcome (which could be continuous, binary, categorical, count variables etc.), and irrespective of the nature (linear or otherwise) of the relationships between the variables. For example, $E(Y|\,\mathbf{C}=\mathbf{c}, X=x, \mathbf{L}=\mathbf{l}, M=m)$ could contain a product term xm, denoting an interaction between exposure and mediator, or any other non-linearities in any of the variables. Thus the controlled direct effect is defined in much more generality than the traditional direct effect, β_x, in (1.1); see limitation "Reliance on linearity" above. Note that (1.9) allows for intermediate confounding variables, also in generality, in the sense that $\mathbf{L}$ could be multivariate, of any type, and the relationship between X, $\mathbf{C}$ and $\mathbf{L}$ could be non-linear. Note too that the derivations in the previous section have made clear that an assumption of no unmeasured confounding between $\mathbf{L}$ and Y is not required, thus the 'infinite regress' suggested in limitation "Exposure-induced confounding" is not in fact an issue.

Having said all this, let us now suppose that there are no intermediate confounders $\mathbf{L}$, and that $E\left(Y \mid \mathbf{C}=\mathbf{c}, X=x, M=m\right)$ is of the simple linear form given in (1.1). Then:

$$
\begin{aligned}
\mathrm{CDE}(m) &= \sum_{\mathbf{c}} E\left(Y \mid \mathbf{C}=\mathbf{c}, X=1, M=m\right) \Pr\left(\mathbf{C}=\mathbf{c}\right) \\
&\quad - \sum_{\mathbf{c}} E\left(Y \mid \mathbf{C}=\mathbf{c}, X=0, M=m\right) \Pr\left(\mathbf{C}=\mathbf{c}\right) \\
&= \sum_{\mathbf{c}} \{E\left(Y \mid \mathbf{C}=\mathbf{c}, X=1, M=m\right) \\
&\quad - E\left(Y \mid \mathbf{C}=\mathbf{c}, X=0, M=m\right)\} \Pr\left(\mathbf{C}=\mathbf{c}\right) \\
&= \sum_{\mathbf{c}} \left\{\left(\beta_0+\beta_x+\beta_m m+\boldsymbol{\beta}_c^T \mathbf{c}\right)-\left(\beta_0+\beta_m m+\boldsymbol{\beta}_c^T \mathbf{c}\right)\right\} \Pr\left(\mathbf{C}=\mathbf{c}\right) \\
&= \sum_{\mathbf{c}} \beta_x \Pr\left(\mathbf{C}=\mathbf{c}\right) \\
&= \beta_x \sum_{\mathbf{c}} \Pr\left(\mathbf{C}=\mathbf{c}\right) \\
&= \beta_x
\end{aligned}
$$

In other words, when there are no intermediate confounders, and the simple linear model for $E\left(Y \mid \mathbf{C}=\mathbf{c}, X=x, M=m\right)$ holds, then under the assumptions given in the previous section, namely no interference for Y, consistency for Y, and CE (i) and (ii), the controlled direct effect is the same for each m, and coincides with the direct effect β_x defined informally at the beginning of the chapter as traditionally used. Thus, the causal inference literature has uncovered unambiguous assumptions under which β_x can be given an interpretation as a direct effect, and has, using counterfactuals, given a possible precise interpretation of this notion of a direct effect, namely as the effect which would remain when fixing the mediator for all at m. In doing so, it allows the generalisation of the notion of a direct effect to non-linear settings. Thus, if we were happy with this prescriptive notion of a direct effect, and were not interested in an indirect effect nor in effect decomposition, what is described in "Identification of the controlled direct effect" would satisfactorily overcome all of the limitations "Reliance on linearity"—"Lack of causal formalism" listed above.

Identification of the natural effects Under the cross-world independence assumption (and hence in the absence of intermediate confounders $\mathbf{L}$), the identification of natural effects follows from the assumptions above using similar steps, except that an additional step is required at the beginning, which is possible under the CWI assumption.

We focus on identifying $E\left\{Y(x, M(x^*))\right\}$, since if this is identified, then by substituting different combinations of 0 and 1 for x and x^*, and taking differences, both the NDE and NIE are also identified.

First, by the law of total expectation, but now conditioning on both $M(x^*)$ and $\mathbf{C} = \mathbf{c}$:

$$E\left\{Y(x, M(x^*))\right\} = \sum_{\mathbf{c},m} E\left\{Y(x, M(x^*))|\mathbf{C} = \mathbf{c}, M(x^*) = m\right\}$$
$$\Pr\left(M(x^*) = m\,|\mathbf{C} = \mathbf{c}\right)\Pr\left(\mathbf{C} = \mathbf{c}\right).$$

In the conditional expectation on the RHS of the above equation, we can replace $Y(x, M(x^*))$ with $Y(x, m)$, since the expectation is taken in a subset for which $M(x^*) = m$, obtaining:

$$E\left\{Y(x, M(x^*))\right\} = \sum_{\mathbf{c},m} E\left\{Y(x, m)|\mathbf{C} = \mathbf{c}, M(x^*) = m\right\}\Pr\left(M(x^*) = m\,|\mathbf{C} = \mathbf{c}\right)$$
$$\Pr\left(\mathbf{C} = \mathbf{c}\right). \tag{1.10}$$

It is at this step that the CWI is used, giving us the license to remove $M(x^*) = m$ from the RHS of the conditional expectation, to give:

$$E\left\{Y(x, M(x^*))\right\} = \sum_{\mathbf{c},m} E\left\{Y(x, m)|\mathbf{C} = \mathbf{c}\right\}\Pr\left(M(x^*) = m\,|\mathbf{C} = \mathbf{c}\right)\Pr\left(\mathbf{C} = \mathbf{c}\right). \tag{1.11}$$

The remainder follows as before. By CE (i):

$$E\left\{Y(x, M(x^*))\right\} = \sum_{\mathbf{c},m} E\left\{Y(x, m)|\mathbf{C} = \mathbf{c}, X = x\right\}$$
$$\Pr\left(M(x^*) = m\,|\mathbf{C} = \mathbf{c}\right)\Pr\left(\mathbf{C} = \mathbf{c}\right).$$

By CE (ii):

$$E\left\{Y(x, M(x^*))\right\} = \sum_{\mathbf{c},m} E\left\{Y(x, m)|\mathbf{C} = \mathbf{c}, X = x, M = m\right\}$$
$$\Pr\left(M(x^*) = m\,|\mathbf{C} = \mathbf{c}\right)\Pr\left(\mathbf{C} = \mathbf{c}\right).$$

By CE (iii):

$$E\left\{Y(x, M(x^*))\right\} = \sum_{\mathbf{c},m} E\left\{Y(x, m)|\mathbf{C} = \mathbf{c}, X = x, M = m\right\}$$
$$\Pr\left(M(x^*) = m\,\middle|\mathbf{C} = \mathbf{c}, X = x^*\right)\Pr\left(\mathbf{C} = \mathbf{c}\right).$$

By consistency for the outcome:

$$E\left\{Y(x, M(x^*))\right\} = \sum_{\mathbf{c},m} E\left(Y|\mathbf{C} = \mathbf{c}, X = x, M = m\right)$$

$$\Pr\left(M(x^*) = m \left| \mathbf{C} = \mathbf{c}, X = x^* \right.\right) \Pr\left(\mathbf{C} = \mathbf{c}\right),$$

and by consistency for the mediator:

$$E\left\{Y(x, M(x^*))\right\} = \sum_{\mathbf{c},m} E\left(Y|\mathbf{C} = \mathbf{c}, X = x, M = m\right)$$
$$\Pr\left(M = m \left| \mathbf{C} = \mathbf{c}, X = x^* \right.\right) \Pr\left(\mathbf{C} = \mathbf{c}\right).$$

Thus, by substituting the appropriate values of 0 or 1 for x and x^*, and taking the appropriate differences:

$$\begin{aligned}
\text{NDE} = &\sum_{\mathbf{c},m} E\left(Y|\mathbf{C} = \mathbf{c}, X = 1, M = m\right) \Pr\left(M = m \left|\mathbf{C} = \mathbf{c}, X = 0\right.\right) \Pr\left(\mathbf{C} = \mathbf{c}\right) \\
&- \sum_{\mathbf{c},m} E\left(Y|\mathbf{C} = \mathbf{c}, X = 0, M = m\right) \Pr\left(M = m \left|\mathbf{C} = \mathbf{c}, X = 0\right.\right) \Pr\left(\mathbf{C} = \mathbf{c}\right) \\
= &\sum_{\mathbf{c},m} \left\{E\left(Y|\mathbf{C} = \mathbf{c}, X = 1, M = m\right) - E\left(Y|\mathbf{C} = \mathbf{c}, X = 0, M = m\right)\right\} \\
&\Pr\left(M = m \left|\mathbf{C} = \mathbf{c}, X = 0\right.\right) \Pr\left(\mathbf{C} = \mathbf{c}\right)
\end{aligned}$$

and

$$\begin{aligned}
\text{NIE} = &\sum_{\mathbf{c},m} E\left(Y|\mathbf{C} = \mathbf{c}, X = 1, M = m\right) \Pr\left(M = m \left|\mathbf{C} = \mathbf{c}, X = 1\right.\right) \Pr\left(\mathbf{C} = \mathbf{c}\right) \\
&- \sum_{\mathbf{c},m} E\left(Y|\mathbf{C} = \mathbf{c}, X = 1, M = m\right) \Pr\left(M = m \left|\mathbf{C} = \mathbf{c}, X = 0\right.\right) \Pr\left(\mathbf{C} = \mathbf{c}\right) \\
= &\sum_{\mathbf{c},m} E\left(Y|\mathbf{C} = \mathbf{c}, X = 1, M = m\right) \\
&\left\{\Pr\left(M = m \left|\mathbf{C} = \mathbf{c}, X = 1\right.\right) - \Pr\left(M = m \left|\mathbf{C} = \mathbf{c}, X = 0\right.\right)\right\} \Pr\left(\mathbf{C} = \mathbf{c}\right).
\end{aligned}$$

The formula above is known as *Pearl's mediation formula*.

Comparison of the NDE with β_x and the NIE with $\alpha_x\beta_m$ Except for limitation "Exposure-induced confounding" concerning intermediate confounding, the two formulae above overcome all the limitations of the traditional approaches, and, unlike the controlled direct effect, they do so for both the direct and indirect effects, in a way that permits effect decomposition. As was pointed out for the CDE, these formulae apply in general, for any type of mediator and outcome variables, and for any (linear or non-linear) relationship between the variables.

However, similar to what we saw before, if (1.1) and (1.3) do hold, together with all the assumptions given in Sect. 1.2.2.3, then the NDE and NIE simplify as follows (note that in the following we adapt the equations to account for the fact that M is continuous):

$$
\begin{aligned}
&\text{NDE} = \\
&\sum_{\mathbf{c}} \int_{m} \{E(Y|\mathbf{C}=\mathbf{c}, X=1, M=m) - E(Y|\mathbf{C}=\mathbf{c}, X=0, M=m)\} \\
&\qquad f_{M|\mathbf{C},X}(m|\mathbf{c},0)\, dm \Pr(\mathbf{C}=\mathbf{c}) \\
&= \sum_{\mathbf{c}} \int_{m} \beta_x f_{M|\mathbf{C},X}(m|\mathbf{c},0)\, dm \Pr(\mathbf{C}=\mathbf{c}) \\
&= \beta_x
\end{aligned}
$$

and

$$
\begin{aligned}
\text{NIE} &= \sum_{\mathbf{c}} \int_{m} E(Y|\mathbf{C}=\mathbf{c}, X=1, M=m) \left\{ f_{M|\mathbf{C},X}(m|\mathbf{c},1) - f_{M|\mathbf{C},X}(m|\mathbf{c},0) \right\} \\
&\qquad dm \Pr(\mathbf{C}=\mathbf{c}) \\
&= \sum_{\mathbf{c}} \int_{m} \left(\beta_0 + \beta_x + \beta_m m + \beta_{\mathbf{c}}^T \mathbf{c}\right) \left\{ f_{M|\mathbf{C},X}(m|\mathbf{c},1) - f_{M|\mathbf{C},X}(m|\mathbf{c},0) \right\} \\
&\qquad dm \Pr(\mathbf{C}=\mathbf{c}) \\
&= \sum_{\mathbf{c}} \int_{m} \beta_m m \left\{ f_{M|\mathbf{C},X}(m|\mathbf{c},1) - f_{M|\mathbf{C},X}(m|\mathbf{c},0) \right\} dm \Pr(\mathbf{C}=\mathbf{c}) \\
&= \sum_{\mathbf{c}} \beta_m \{E(M|\mathbf{C}=\mathbf{c}, X=1) - E(M|\mathbf{C}=\mathbf{c}, X=0)\} \Pr(\mathbf{C}=\mathbf{c}) \\
&= \beta_m \alpha_x
\end{aligned}
$$

Again therefore, when there are no intermediate confounders, and the simple linear models for $E(Y|\mathbf{C}=\mathbf{c}, X=x, M=m)$ and $E(M|\mathbf{C}=\mathbf{c}, X=x)$ hold, then under the assumptions given in Sect. 1.2.2.3, namely no interference for Y and M, consistency for Y and M, conditional exchangeability (i), (ii) and (iii), and the cross-world independent assumption, the natural direct effect coincides with β_x (which as we have already noted coincides with the CDE for each m), and the natural indirect effect coincides with $\alpha_x\beta_m = \gamma_x - \beta_x$. Thus, the causal inference literature has uncovered unambiguous assumptions under which these informal direct and indirect effects can be given an interpretation as direct and indirect effects, and, using counterfactuals, given another possible precise interpretation of these notions, thereby allowing the effects to be defined in non-linear settings. If we were happy to make the strong cross-world independence assumption, ruling out intermediate confounders, what is described above would satisfactorily overcome limitations "Reliance on linearity", "M–Y confounding" and "Lack of causal formalism" listed above.

Identification of the interventional effects Even if we were happy to assume that there are no intermediate confounders, going from (1.10) to (1.11) above is only permitted under the CWI assumption, which as we have already noted is a stronger assumption. One way of intuitively understanding the alternative interventional effects is that they avoid having to make the step from (1.10) to (1.11) by changing the estimand to that which is equal to (1.11), irrespective of whether or not the CWI assumption holds.

The identification steps then follow in a similar way to those in section "Identification of the natural effects", except that intermediate confounders **L** are now permitted, and thus are included as shown below.

By definition (i.e. not by assumption), we have that:

$$E\left\{Y\left(x, M^*_{x^*|\mathbf{C}}\right)\right\} = \sum_{\mathbf{c},m} E\left\{Y(x,m)|\mathbf{C}=\mathbf{c}\right\} \Pr\left(M(x^*)=m\,|\mathbf{C}=\mathbf{c}\right) \Pr\left(\mathbf{C}=\mathbf{c}\right).$$

Then by CE (i):

$$E\left\{Y\left(x, M^*_{x^*|\mathbf{C}}\right)\right\} = \sum_{\mathbf{c},m} E\left\{Y(x,m)|\mathbf{C}=\mathbf{c}, X=x\right\} \Pr\left(M(x^*)=m\,|\mathbf{C}=\mathbf{c}\right) \Pr\left(\mathbf{C}=\mathbf{c}\right).$$

By the law of total expectations, as was applied in section "Identification of the controlled direct effect":

$$E\left\{Y\left(x, M^*_{x^*|\mathbf{C}}\right)\right\} = \sum_{\mathbf{c},\mathbf{l},m} E\left\{Y(x,m)|\mathbf{C}=\mathbf{c}, X=x, \mathbf{L}=\mathbf{l}\right\} \Pr\left(\mathbf{L}=\mathbf{l}\,|\mathbf{C}=\mathbf{c}, X=x\right)$$
$$\Pr\left(M(x^*)=m\,|\mathbf{C}=\mathbf{c}\right) \Pr\left(\mathbf{C}=\mathbf{c}\right).$$

By CE (ii):

$$E\left\{Y\left(x, M^*_{x^*|\mathbf{C}}\right)\right\} = \sum_{\mathbf{c},\mathbf{l},m} E\left\{Y(x,m)|\mathbf{C}=\mathbf{c}, X=x, \mathbf{L}=\mathbf{l}, M=m\right\} \Pr\left(\mathbf{L}=\mathbf{l}\,|\mathbf{C}=\mathbf{c}, X=x\right)$$
$$\Pr\left(M(x^*)=m\,|\mathbf{C}=\mathbf{c}\right) \Pr\left(\mathbf{C}=\mathbf{c}\right).$$

By CE (iii):

$$E\left\{Y\left(x, M^*_{x^*|\mathbf{C}}\right)\right\} = \sum_{\mathbf{c},\mathbf{l},m} E\left\{Y(x,m)|\mathbf{C}=\mathbf{c}, X=x, \mathbf{L}=\mathbf{l}, M=m\right\} \Pr\left(\mathbf{L}=\mathbf{l}\,|\mathbf{C}=\mathbf{c}, X=x\right)$$
$$\Pr\left(M(x^*)=m\,|\mathbf{C}=\mathbf{c}, X=x\right) \Pr\left(\mathbf{C}=\mathbf{c}\right).$$

And finally by consistency for the mediator and the outcome:

$$E\left\{Y\left(x, M^*_{x^*|\mathbf{C}}\right)\right\} = \sum_{\mathbf{c},\mathbf{l},m} E\left\{Y|\mathbf{C}=\mathbf{c}, X=x, \mathbf{L}=\mathbf{l}, M=m\right\} \Pr\left(\mathbf{L}=\mathbf{l}\,|\mathbf{C}=\mathbf{c}, X=x\right)$$
$$\Pr\left(M=m\,|\mathbf{C}=\mathbf{c}, X=x\right) \Pr\left(\mathbf{C}=\mathbf{c}\right).$$

Thus, by substituting the appropriate values of 0 or 1 for x and x^*, and taking the appropriate differences:

$$\begin{aligned}
\text{RIA-NDE} &= \sum_{\mathbf{c},\mathbf{l},m} E\left(Y|\mathbf{C}=\mathbf{c}, X=1, \mathbf{L}=\mathbf{l}, M=m\right) \Pr\left(\mathbf{L}=\mathbf{l}\,|\mathbf{C}=\mathbf{c}, X=1\right) \\
&\qquad \Pr\left(M=m\,|\mathbf{C}=\mathbf{c}, X=0\right) \Pr\left(\mathbf{C}=\mathbf{c}\right) \\
&\quad - \sum_{\mathbf{c},\mathbf{l},m} E\left(Y|\mathbf{C}=\mathbf{c}, X=0, \mathbf{L}=\mathbf{l}, M=m\right) \Pr\left(\mathbf{L}=\mathbf{l}\,|\mathbf{C}=\mathbf{c}, X=0\right) \\
&\qquad \Pr\left(M=m\,|\mathbf{C}=\mathbf{c}, X=0\right) \Pr\left(\mathbf{C}=\mathbf{c}\right) \\
&= \sum_{\mathbf{c},\mathbf{l},m} \{E\left(Y|\mathbf{C}=\mathbf{c}, X=1, \mathbf{L}=\mathbf{l}, M=m\right) \Pr\left(\mathbf{L}=\mathbf{l}\,|\mathbf{C}=\mathbf{c}, X=1\right) \\
&\quad - E\left(Y|\mathbf{C}=\mathbf{c}, X=0, \mathbf{L}=\mathbf{l}, M=m\right) \Pr\left(\mathbf{L}=\mathbf{l}\,|\mathbf{C}=\mathbf{c}, X=0\right)\} \\
&\qquad \Pr\left(M=m\,|\mathbf{C}=\mathbf{c}, X=0\right) \Pr\left(\mathbf{C}=\mathbf{c}\right)
\end{aligned}$$

and

$$\begin{aligned}
\text{RIA-NIE} &= \sum_{\mathbf{c},\mathbf{l},m} E\left(Y|\mathbf{C}=\mathbf{c}, X=1, \mathbf{L}=\mathbf{l}, M=m\right) \Pr\left(\mathbf{L}=\mathbf{l}\,|\mathbf{C}=\mathbf{c}, X=1\right) \\
&\qquad \Pr\left(M=m\,|\mathbf{C}=\mathbf{c}, X=1\right) \Pr\left(\mathbf{C}=\mathbf{c}\right) \\
&\quad - \sum_{\mathbf{c},\mathbf{l},m} E\left(Y|\mathbf{C}=\mathbf{c}, X=1, \mathbf{L}=\mathbf{l}, M=m\right) \\
&\qquad \Pr\left(\mathbf{L}=\mathbf{l}\,|\mathbf{C}=\mathbf{c}, X=1\right) \Pr\left(M=m\,|\mathbf{C}=\mathbf{c}, X=0\right) \Pr\left(\mathbf{C}=\mathbf{c}\right) \\
&= \sum_{\mathbf{c},\mathbf{l},m} E\left(Y|\mathbf{C}=\mathbf{c}, X=1, \mathbf{L}=\mathbf{l}, M=m\right) \Pr\left(\mathbf{L}=\mathbf{l}\,|\mathbf{C}=\mathbf{c}, X=1\right) \\
&\qquad \{\Pr\left(M=m\,|\mathbf{C}=\mathbf{c}, X=1\right) - \Pr\left(M=m\,|\mathbf{C}=\mathbf{c}, X=0\right)\} \Pr\left(\mathbf{C}=\mathbf{c}\right)
\end{aligned}$$

1.2.2.5 Estimation and Software

To estimate the effects above, the most obvious approach is to fit separate regression models for each conditional expectation or probability (or density) in the right hand side of the identification equations, estimate the parameters of these models from the data (typically by ML), use these estimates to calculate predicted expectations and probabilities (or densities), and then to plug them into the equations above (*plug-in estimation*). As we have noted, there is no restriction on how these models are specified, as long as it is possible to predict the relevant conditional expectations and probabilities (or densities) from them, so that these may be plugged in; interactions and other non-linearities can be included, as well as non-identity link functions.

The asymptotic (i.e. in large samples) unbiasedness of the resulting plug-in estimators then relies on the correct specification of the contributing conditional expectations and probabilities (in addition to all relevant identifying assumptions above). In the presence of multi-dimensional intermediate confounders **L**, this amounts to a very large number of additional parametric assumptions.

Standard errors can sometimes be approximated via the delta method, otherwise the bootstrap can be used Efron and Tibshirani (1993).

The evaluation of the sums (and/or integrals) involved in the identifying equations may become cumbersome or even analytically intractable, depending on the form and complexity of the contributing models. Although the associated plug-in estimators have been analytically derived for many combinations of models Valeri and VanderWeele (2013), Monte Carlo (MC) simulation is used for more complex settings.

Routines for the Implementation of these approaches in statistical software packages to estimate CDE and NDE/NIE in the absence of intermediate confounders are available, e.g. (Emsley, liu, Dunn, Valeri, & VanderWeele, 2014; Muthén, 2011, Tingley, Yamamoto, Hirose, Keele, & Imai, 2011; Valeri & VanderWeele, 2013). In the presence of intermediate confounders the CDE and RIA-NDE and RIA-NIE can be estimated using `gformula` in Stata Daniel, De Stavola, and Cousens (2011).

Several alternative approaches have been proposed that do not require the specification of parametric models for all the components of the identifying equations. In particular, where relevant, these alternatives do away with the need to specify the joint density of the intermediate confounders given X and $\mathbf{C}$. They include inverse probability weighting of marginal structural models for the potential outcomes VanderWeele (2009a) or for the natural effects Lange et al. (2012), inverse odds ratio weighting (IORW) Tchetgen Tchetgen and VanderWeele (2014), sequential g-estimation Vansteelandt and Joffe (2014), and imputation-based estimation Vansteelandt et al. (2012), among others.

1.3 Survival Outcomes

In several life course investigations the outcome of interest is the timing of an event. Let T denote such a variable, $S(t) = Pr(T > t)$ the corresponding survival probability function, and $\lambda(t)$ the hazard rate at time t, i.e. the instantaneous rate of the event conditional on survival up to time t. In most such settings effect measures of an exposure are expressed in terms of hazard ratios or hazard differences, although in some contexts the focus is on some other aspects of the distribution of T, for example its mean, $E(T)$, or the cumulative risk of the event by time t, $Pr(T \leq t) = 1 - S(t)$. When concerned with mediation analysis we might therefore wish to decompose the total effect of an exposure on any of these scales.

Due to the inherent non-linearities involved when sensibly modelling hazards and survivor functions, it is perhaps not surprising in the light of our discussions so far, that the majority of proposals for mediation analysis for time to event data have been from the causal inference literature (Lange & Hansen, 2011; Luo & Geng, 2016; Martinussen & Vansteelandt, 2013; Martinussen, Vansteelandt, Gerster, & Hjelmborg, 2011; Tchetgen Tchetgen, 2011; VanderWeele, 2011) (with some exceptions, see for example Aalen, 2012; Fosen, Ferkingstad, Borgan, & Aalen, 2006; Gelfand, MacKinnon, De Rubeis, & Baraldi, 2016; Tein & MacKinnon, 2003) and therefore involving aspects of the distribution of *potential* survival times. For example, the counterfactual hazard function $\lambda_{T(x,M(x^*))}(t)$ is used to denote the hypothetical hazard function for the event of interest were the exposure to be set to x and the mediator to the value it would have attained had the exposure been set to x^*.

Natural direct and indirect effects defined as hazard ratios (HR) are then given by VanderWeele (2015, 2011):

$$\text{NDE}^{\text{HR}}(t) = \frac{\lambda_{T(1,M(0))}(t)}{\lambda_{T(0,M(0))}(t)}, \qquad \text{NIE}^{\text{HR}}(t) = \frac{\lambda_{T(1,M(1))}(t)}{\lambda_{T(1,M(0))}(t)}.$$

Alternatively natural mediation effects expressed as mean survival time ratios (MR) are VanderWeele (2015, 2011):

$$\text{NDE}^{\text{MR}} = \frac{E\{T(1, M(0))\}}{E\{T(0, M(0))\}}, \qquad \text{NIE}^{\text{MR}} = \frac{E\{T(1, M(1))\}}{E\{T(1, M(0))\}}.$$

As discussed in Sect. 1.2.2, estimating mediation effects relies on structural and parametric assumptions. The structural assumptions are as before (with T in place of Y), but the parametric models for T will typically be of a different form from the ones considered for Y above.

It may be assumed, for example, that T follows an accelerated failure time (AFT) model, such as:

$$\log(T) = \theta_0 + \theta_x X + \theta_m M + \theta_{xm} XM + \boldsymbol{\theta}_c^T \mathbf{C} + \epsilon_T$$

where ϵ_T is an error term following an extreme value distribution VanderWeele (2015, 2011). If this model is correctly specified and if M given X and $\mathbf{C}$ is normally distributed with mean as defined in (1.3) and standard deviation σ_m, VanderWeele (2015, 2011) showed that the natural effects expressed as mean survival time ratios are identified by:

$$\begin{aligned}\text{NDE}^{\text{MR}} &= \exp\left\{\theta_x + \theta_{xm}\left(\alpha_0 + \alpha_x X + \boldsymbol{\alpha}_c^T \mathbf{C} + \theta_m \sigma_m^2\right) + 0.5\theta_{xm}^2 \sigma_m^2\right\} \\ \text{NIE}^{\text{MR}} &= \exp\left(\theta_m \alpha_x + \theta_{xm} \alpha_x\right).\end{aligned}$$

Note that in the absence of an X–M interaction, these expressions closely resemble the results shown in Sect. 1.2.1.

Alternatively, we may assume that T follows a proportional hazards (PH) model, such as:

$$\lambda(t|X, M, \mathbf{C}) = \lambda_0(t) \exp\left(\delta_x X + \delta_m M + \delta_{xm} XM + \boldsymbol{\delta}_c^T \mathbf{C}\right) \tag{1.12}$$

If this and the model for M described above are correctly specified *and* if the event of interest is rare, VanderWeele (2015, 2011) showed that the natural effects expressed as HRs are approximately identified by:

$$\begin{aligned} \text{NDE}^{\text{HR}} &= \exp\left(\delta_x + \delta_{xm}\left(\alpha_0 + \alpha_x X + \boldsymbol{\alpha}_c^T \mathbf{C} + \delta_m \sigma_m^2\right) + 0.5\delta_{xm}^2 \sigma_m^2\right) \\ \text{NIE}^{\text{HR}} &= \exp\left(\delta_m \alpha_x + \delta_{xm} \alpha_x\right). \end{aligned} \tag{1.13}$$

Extensions of these expressions for PH models such as (1.12) are available for settings where M is binary VanderWeele (2011).

Yet another alternative is to assume an additive hazards model for T, such as:

$$\lambda\left(t|X, M, \mathbf{C}\right) = \lambda_0^{\dagger}\left(t\right) + \delta_x^{\dagger}\left(t\right) X + \delta_m^{\dagger}\left(t\right) M + \boldsymbol{\delta}_c^{\dagger T}\left(t\right) \mathbf{C}. \tag{1.14}$$

If this model is correctly specified and M given X and $\mathbf{C}$ is normally distributed with mean as described in (1.3) and constant variance, natural direct and indirect effects expressed as differences in hazards can be derived by applying the product method described in Sect. 1.2.1 at every event time. This is an example of dynamic path analysis (Fosen et al., 2006; Lange & Hansen, 2011) which, under the assumptions stated, does not require the event to be rare, unlike the results for hazard ratios.

When the coefficients in model (1.14) are constant, the partitioning of natural effects in terms of hazard differences (HD) is given in closed form (Lange & Hansen, 2011; Nemes et al., 2013; VanderWeele, 2015) as:

$$\begin{aligned} \text{NDE}^{\text{HD}} &= \delta_x^{\dagger} \\ \text{NIE}^{\text{HD}} &= \delta_m^{\dagger} \alpha_x. \end{aligned} \tag{1.15}$$

Estimation of these effects can then be achieved using plug-in estimation as described in Sects. 1.2.1 and 1.2.2.5. A dedicated SAS macro ia available to implement mediation analysis on the HR or MR scales Valeri and VanderWeele (2015), while Lange and Hansen (2011) gives the R code for mediation analysis on the HD scale.

1.4 Example

We now illustrate an application of mediation analysis to a simulated dataset, sufficiently large so as to render negligible any finite sample variation in the results from different analyses. Although simulated and in some aspects simplified for illustrative purposes, the data still reflect a combination of realistic features we have encountered in various applications in our own experience as well as in the literature. Details of the data generation are given in the Web Appendix.

1.4.1 Context

Suppose a study has identified a socio-economic disparity in childhood respiratory diseases that is widening over time. Suppose too that one possible explanation for this observed trend is the corresponding increase in medically-induced preterm deliveries (MIPD) over a similar period, which is thought to be particularly pronounced in mothers of low socio-economic position (SEP). As part of an investigation into this, suppose that a study is conducted to explore the mediating role of MIPD in the effect of low maternal SEP on her child's lung function at 12 months.

1.4.2 Data and Possible Causal Diagram

The simulated data contain information on 1,000,000 singleton infants whose lung function (FEV) was recorded at 12 months (with the values rescaled to have mean 0 and standard deviation 1) as well as on maternal SEP (dichotomised, for simplicity, as 1 = low or 0 = high) and whether or not the delivery was medically-induced at preterm (MIPD, 1 = yes, 0 = no). Also available is information on maternal pre-pregnancy BMI (also dichotomised for simplicity as 0=non-obese for $<30\,\text{kg/m}^2$ and 1 = obese for $\geq 30\,\text{kg/m}^2$), the infant's year of birth (between 1998 and 2000) and sex. In reality, more covariate information is likely to be available, and a finer categorisation of SEP and maternal body size would also be used, but for simplicity we will use just these variables and in these forms for the duration of this illustration.

Simple exploration of the data reveals that the children are equally balanced between boys and girls and that about 36% of the mothers have low SEP. These mothers also are more frequently obese (24.7% vs. 18.5%), and their infants are more frequently born preterm by medical intervention (13.4% vs. 9.5%) than infants of mothers with high SEP. These children have lower average lung function than children whose mothers are high SEP (mean difference: 0.18 SD). The average difference in lung function by MIPD is more pronounced (0.66 SD lower for those whose delivery was medically induced).

If we were prepared to assume that the measured confounders are sufficient to adjust for all confounding of the exposure–mediator, mediator–outcome and exposure–outcome relationships, then a possible causal diagram would be that shown in Fig. 1.6. Note that according to this diagram, year of birth and sex are confounders not affected by exposure (**C**), and maternal obesity is a confounder of mediator and outcome potentially affected by the exposure, i.e. an intermediate confounder (L). The unmeasured common cause U of year of birth and maternal SEP is included to allow for the fact that there might be changes in maternal SEP over time, and hence that the two variables are associated, even though neither causes the other.

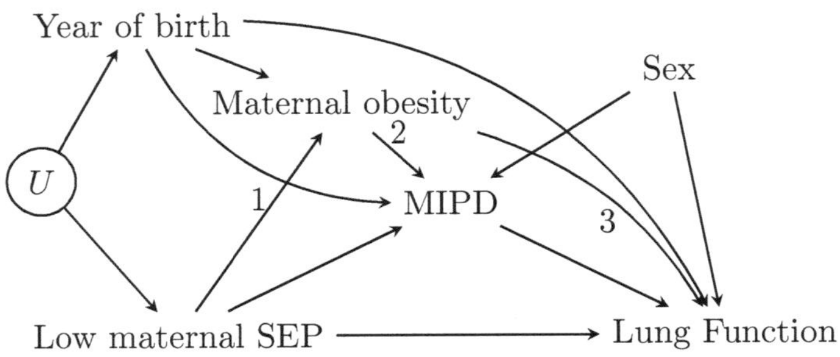

Fig. 1.6 Causal diagram for the simulated example. Note that the numbers attached to the arrows are referred to in the text

1.4.3 Possible Estimands

In this example, the two controlled direct effects, CDE(0) and CDE(1), would capture the effect (on lung function at 12 months) of changing maternal SEP for all mothers, whilst either eradicating MIPD or making it universal. The latter, CDE(1), is very unlikely to be of interest, and even the former, due to the necessity of MIPD in some circumstances, is somewhat unrealistic.

For this reason, as well as due to our interest in the indirect effect mediated by MIPD, and in effect decomposition, we focus on the natural direct and indirect effects. The NDE captures the effect (on lung function at 12 months) of changing maternal SEP for all mothers, whilst setting each mother's MIPD status to the level at which it would have been had the mother been of high SEP. The NIE then captures the effect (on lung function at 12 months) of changing each mother's MIPD status from what it would have been had the mother been of high SEP to what it would have been had she been of low SEP, whilst setting maternal SEP to low for all mothers.

As discussed, the assumptions under which the NDE and NIE can be identified are exceptionally strong, and are known to be violated in the presence of intermediate confounders, such as maternal obesity in this example. For this reason, we will also focus on the randomised intervention analogues of the NDE and NIE. In this example, the RIA-NDE captures the effect (on lung function at 12 months) of changing maternal SEP for all mothers, whilst setting each mother's MIPD status to a random draw from the conditional counterfactual distribution of MIPD given baseline confounders, in a hypothetical world in which all mothers are of high SEP. The RIA-NIE captures the effect (on lung function at 12 months) of changing each mother's MIPD status from a draw from the conditional counterfactual distribution of MIPD given baseline confounders had all mothers been of high SEP to a draw from the corresponding conditional counterfactual distribution had all women been of low SEP, whilst setting maternal SEP to low for all mothers.

1.4.4 Methods and Model Choices

For completeness, we start by implementing the path analysis approach. Since our mediator (MIPD) is binary, the difference method is more natural.[7] The difference method constrains us to fitting quite simple models, corresponding to (1.1) and (1.2) in Sect. 1.2.1. The only flexibility afforded to us in choosing the forms of (1.1) and (1.2) is in how we include the background confounders $\mathbf{C}$ in the models; X must enter as a single term in both (1.1) and (1.2), which entails not including the product of X and M in (1.1), and thus being unable to allow for an exposure–mediator interaction. We choose to fit as flexible a pair of models as is allowed under these contraints: they contain all background confounders as binary/categorical variables, with all possible (two-way and higher-order) interactions between them, together with a main effect of X, and additionally a main effect of M and all (two-way and higher-order) interactions between M and $\mathbf{C}$ in (1.1). The chosen models are shown in the Web Appendix.

As we have discussed, there is no way of incorporating the intermediate confounder L (maternal obesity) satisfactorily when using the difference method, and thus we consider two (sub-optimal) strategies, namely first ignoring L entirely, and second treating L as another background confounder (and thus including all two-way and higher-order interactions between L and $\mathbf{C}$ and L and M, where applicable). The first strategy would be invalid if both arrows 2 and 3 in Fig. 1.6 were non-null, and the second strategy would be invalid if arrow 1 were non-null. When all three arrows are non-null, the relative performance of the two strategies will depend on the strengths of 1, 2 and 3 relative to each other (as well as relative to the strengths of other arrows in the diagram), but we would not expect either to be valid. A hybrid option would be to treat L as a background confounder in model (1.1) but to ignore it in model (1.2); we don't consider this option further in the interest of brevity.

The parameters of the two models are estimated by OLS and the indirect effect derived as the difference between the two coefficients of X as discussed in Sect. 1.2.1. All standard errors are obtained using the non-parametric bootstrap (with 1,000) bootstrap samples.

If the diagram in Fig. 1.6 were correct, and if at least one of arrows 2 or 3 were null and, furthermore, if the simple parametric models described above were correctly specified, i.e. if they were correct in omitting product terms between X and, where relevant, M, L and $\mathbf{C}$, then, under the additional technical assumptions of no interference and consistency, we would be able to interpret the total, direct and indirect effect estimates resulting from the difference method under the first strategy causally. Under these assumptions, the two controlled direct effects would be equal, and both would be equal to the randomised interventional analogue of the natural direct effect and thus the estimate $\hat{\beta}_x$ could be interpreted in any of these ways; if, additionally, the cross-world independence assumption is true then the same estimate can be interpreted as the natural direct effect. Likewise, under all the assumptions

[7] Although note that identical results would be obtained using the product method were we to use a linear probability model for the binary mediator.

above, in addition to the cross-world independence assumption, our estimate $\hat{\gamma}_x - \hat{\beta}_x$ of the indirect effect can be interpreted as both the natural indirect effect and its randomised interventional analogue, since these too would coincide. Similarly, if the same assumptions were to hold except that arrow 1 were null (rather than arrows 2 or 3), then the same could be said of the difference method under the second strategy.

However, we ideally wish to make fewer parametric assumptions, we wish to acknowledge L's role as an intermediate confounder, and we wish to avoid making the CWI assumption. Thus we adopt a third strategy: we use the plug-in approach described in Sect. 1.2.2.4, with the cumbersome summations circumvented by using Monte Carlo simulation. The large sample size, coupled with the relatively small number of variables, all of which are discrete except for the outcome, allows us to be entirely non-parametric in our associational models. That is, each model contains all possible two-way, three-way, four-way and five-way interactions (where applicable) and thus is saturated and—unlike what we could do using the difference method—guaranteed not to be misspecified. Under no parametric assumptions, therefore, the total, overall, CDE(0), CDE(1), RIA-NDE and RIA-NIE effects that we estimate can be given the appropriate interpretation under the technical and structural assumptions given in Sect. 1.2.2.3. If, in addition, we could make the cross-world independence assumption, or one of the slightly weaker alternatives, the RIA effects could also be interpreted as the NDE and NIE, respectively. But as we have said, given that maternal obesity is plausibly a non-trivial intermediate confounder, these additional assumptions are unlikely to hold.

We again use the non-parametric bootstrap to estimate standard errors.

Stata code for fitting all these analyses is included in the Web Appendix.

1.4.5 Results

The results are shown in Table 1.1. For completeness, we have performed the full plug-in estimation procedure with MC simulation for the situations in which we ignore L or treat it as a background confounder, as well as the situation in which we treat it as an intermediate confounder, even though we would believe the last to be the best of the three. Thus, the results in bold are the ones that we consider most carefully.

First note that treating L as a background confounder seems to be more problematic in this scenario than ignoring it completely. Even the estimate of the total effect is badly affected, since we are adjusting for a variable, maternal obesity, that lies on a strong causal pathway from exposure to outcome. Ignoring L does not seem as problematic, although we see small biases, as we discuss further below. This is since the confounding effect of maternal obesity on the relationship between MIPD and lung function is not very strong in this example.

Second, we note that the two controlled direct effects are quite different from one another, pointing to a non-negligible interaction between maternal low SEP and

Table 1.1 Estimated mediation effects for the example

	Ignoring L		Treating L as a background confounder		Treating L as an intermediate confounder	
	Estimate	SE	Estimate	SE	Estimate	SE
Difference method:						
Total	**−0.158**	(0.0020)	**−0.100**	(0.0019)	−0.158	(0.0020)
Direct	**−0.129**	(0.0019)	**−0.083**	(0.0018)	–	–
Indirect	**−0.029**	(0.0005)	**−0.017**	(0.0004)	–	–
Non-parametric plug-in estimation using MC simulation:						
Total	−0.160	(0.0020)	−0.098	(0.0019)	**−0.160**	(0.0020)
CDE(0)	−0.097	(0.0021)	−0.053	(0.0020)	**−0.109**	(0.0022)
CDE(1)	−0.380	(0.0066)	−0.304	(0.0066)	**−0.360**	(0.0065)
Overall	−0.160	(0.0021)	−0.099	(0.0027)	**−0.162**	(0.0032)
RIA-NDE	−0.123	(0.0020)	−0.078	(0.0028)	**−0.135**	(0.0037)
RIA-NIE	−0.037	(0.0007)	−0.021	(0.0006)	**−0.026**	(0.0009)

MIPD in their effect on lung function. The harmful effect of MIPD is stronger in the children born to mothers of a low SEP.

Third, the overall and total effects are not so different from each other, which points to the cross-world assumption not being too badly violated (presumably, again, since maternal obesity is not a particularly strong confounder). The RIA-NDE is between the CDE(0) and CDE(1), but is closer to the CDE(0), which is to be expected since the prevalence of the mediator is quite low.

We also note that, in this example, correctly treating L as an intermediate confounder leads to direct effect estimates that are further from the null than the other two strategies. It is perhaps instructive to understand the direction of this change. Low maternal SEP and maternal obesity both increase the risk of MIPD, and so when we adjust for M in (1.1), we induce an additional negative association between low maternal SEP and maternal obesity, which, when we ignore obesity in this model, is not removed. Thus the positive effect of maternal low SEP on obesity is reduced. Consequently, the negative effect of low SEP on lung function, which contributes to the direct effect, is reduced in magnitude, and thus the magnitude of the direct effect overall is underestimated. Alternatively, if we do adjust for L, but as a background confounder, then we block this induced negative association between low SEP and MIPD, but we also eliminate the portion of the direct negative effect of low SEP on lung function that is via maternal obesity, also leading to the magnitude of the direct effect being underestimated.

We have compared horizontally across the table to see the impact of incorrectly allowing for the intermediate confounder. Likewise, by looking vertically down the table, and comparing the estimates obtained using the difference method with the non-parametric plug-in estimation, we see that the effect of parametric model misspecification is not too severe in the difference method in this example. Indeed, even the fact that the difference method fails to allow for a strong X–M interaction has not affected the estimate of the direct effect too badly, if one were to interpret it as an estimate of the RIA-NDE.

It is important to point out that all the observations above are particular to this example and the way in which the data were simulated, and we would expect different examples and setups to lead to different magnitudes and directions of discrepancies between various methods and model choices.

From a substantive point of view, we would conclude from these analyses that, under the assumptions that year of birth is sufficient to control for confounding of low maternal SEP and lung function, and of low maternal SEP and MIPD, and that year of birth, sex and maternal obesity are sufficient to control for confounding of MIPD and lung function, within levels of low maternal SEP, together with the technical assumptions of no interference and consistency, that there is a harmful impact of low maternal SEP on childhood lung function at age 12 months, of around 0.16 SD, with around 17% of this effect being mediated by medically-induced preterm delivery. This would lend support to the hypothesis that the increasing trend of MIPD amongst low SEP mothers partly explains the increase in socioeconomic disparity in childhood lung function, but it would also suggest that there are other important explanations for this trend.

1.5 Concluding Thoughts

In this chapter, we have attempted to give a thorough but accessible introduction to the field of causal mediation analysis and how it relates to more traditional approaches such as path analysis. In particular we have reviewed the assumptions implicit in the traditional approach for the desired interpretation of mediation effects to be justified, and how many of these are relaxed when adopting the more flexible counterfactual-based approach. We have highlighted particular aspects, such as intermediate confounding and survival outcomes, which are particularly pertinent in life course investigations. Mediation analysis is a subject fraught with pitfalls and interpretational and analytic subtleties, and this is a consequence of the fact that mediation analysis is not as intuitive as it might at first sight seem as soon as there are non-linearities in the relationships involved. However, the work done in the field of causal mediation analysis has vastly broadened the scope of the sorts of questions that can be addressed, and the models and methods that can be fitted and used. The inherent mathematical complexities will always underlie these approaches; however, as more applications appear in the literature, and as more software packages are developed, we envisage that these methods will increasingly be used by applied researchers in life course epidemiology and other disciplines.

Inevitably, there are many other developments that we were forced to omit from this chapter in the interest of brevity. For a comprehensive account of the subject we again refer readers to Tyler VanderWeele's recent book VanderWeele (2015). In particular, a challenging but important area in which much progress has recently been made is on extending the material presented in this chapter to problems with multiple mediators of interest (Avin, Shpitser, & Pearl, 2005; Daniel et al., 2015; Nguyen, Osypuk, Schmidt, Glymour, & Tchetgen Tchetgen, 2015; Tchetgen Tchetgen, 2013; VanderWeele et al., 2014; Vansteelandt & Daniel, 2016). These developments are closely related to methods for overcoming intermediate confounding, with interventional effects again proving useful.

In our illustrative example, we used saturated associational models so that parametric model misspecification was not a risk. However, in settings with more variables and/or a smaller sample size, such non-parametric estimation would soon run into the so-called curse of dimensionality problem. In practice, parametric smoothing choices are then typically made, but these have the dissatisfaction of being somewhat arbitrary, of leading to bias when incorrect and to invalid inferences when the choices are based on multiple candidate models (and results), with the danger of further bias due to cherry-picking. In the light of these limitations, a promising alternative, principled approach to data-adaptive inference is that offered by targeted minimum loss based estimation (TMLE) using the ensemble of machine learning algorithms known as the superlearner (van der Laan & Rose, 2011; Zheng & van der Laan, 2012). As the nature of observational datasets gets larger and more complex, and the mediation questions increasingly demanding, e.g. based on high-dimensional multiple mediators, we envisage that principled data-adaptive estimation will become increasingly important within causal mediation analysis.

References

Aalen, O. O. (2012). Armitage lecture 2010: Understanding treatment effects: The value of integrating longitudinal data and survival analysis. *Statistics in Medicine, 31*(18), 1903–1917.

Avin, C., Shpitser, I., Pearl, J. (2005). *Identifiability of Pathspecific Effects in Proceedings of the 19th Joint Conference on Artificial Intelligence.*

Baron, R. M., & Kenny, D. A. (1986). The moderator-mediator variable distinction in social psychological research: Conceptual, strategic, and statistical considerations. *Journal of Personality and Social Psychology, 51*(6), 1173–1182.

Bartoli, F., Crocamo, C., Gennaro, G. M., Castagna, G., Trotta, G., Clerici, M., et al. (2016). Exploring the association between bipolar disorder and uric acid: A mediation analysis. *Journal of Psychosomatic Research, 84*, 56–59.

Benedum, C. M., Yazdy, M. M., Parker, S. E., Mitchell, A. A., & Werler, M. M. (2016). Association of clomiphene and assisted reproductive technologies with the risk of neural tube defects. *American Journal of Epidemiology, 183*, 977987.

Biarnes, M., Arias, L., Alonso, J., & Garcia, M. (2015). Increased fundus autouorescence and progression of geographic atrophy secondary to age-related macular degeneration: The gain study. *American Journal of Ophthalmology, 160*, 34–353.

Bollen, K. A. (1989). *Structural equations with latent variables*. New York: Wiley.

Bollen, K. A., & Pearl, J. (2013). Eight myths about causality and structural equation models. In S.L. Morgan (Ed.), *Handbook of causal analysis for social research* (pp. 301–328). Springer.

Burgess, S., Daniel, R. M., Butterworth, A. S., Thompson, S. G. (2015). The EPIC-InterAct Consortium. Network mendelian randomization: using genetic variants as instrumental variables to investigate mediation in causal pathways. *International Journal of Epidemiology, 44*, 484–495 (2015).

Chen, Y.-H., Mukherjee, B., Ferguson, K. K., Meeker, J. D., & VanderWeele, T. J. (2016). Mediation formula for a binary outcome and a time-varying exposure and mediator, accounting for possible exposure-mediator interaction. *American Journal of Epidemiology, 184*, 157159.

Chen, B., & Pearl, J. (2013). Regression and causation: A critical examination of econometrics textbooks. *Real-World Economics Review, 65*, 2–20.

Cole, S. R., & Frangakis, C. E. (2009). The consistency statement in causal inference: A definition or an assumption? *Epidemiology, 20*(1), 3–5.

Cole, S. R., & Hernán, M. A. (2002). Fallibility in estimating direct effects. *International Journal of Epidemiology, 31*, 163–165.

Cox, D. R. (1958). *Planning of experiments*. New York: Wiley.

Daniel, R. M., De Stavola, B. L., & Vansteelandt, S. (in press). The formal approach to quantitative causal inference in epidemiology: misguided or misrepresented? *International Journal of Epidemiology.*

Daniel, R. M., De Stavola, B. L., & Cousens, S. N. (2011). gformula: Estimating causal effects in the presence of time-varying confounding or mediation using the g-computation formula. *The Stata Journal, 11*(4), 479–517.

Daniel, R. M., De Stavola, B. L., Cousens, S., & Vansteelandt, S. (2015). Causal mediation analysis with multiple causally-ordered mediators. *Biometrics, 71*, 1–14.

De Stavola, B. L., Daniel, R. M., Ploubidis, G. B., & Micali, N. (2015). Mediation analysis with intermediate confounding: structural equation modeling viewed through the causal inference lens. *American Journal of Epidemiology, 181*, 64–80.

Didelez, V., Dawid P., & Geneletti, S. (2006). Direct and indirect effects of sequential treatments. In *Proceedings of the 22nd Annual Conference on Uncertainty in Artifical Intelligence,* 138–146.

Efron, B., & Tibshirani, R. J. (1993). *An introduction to the bootstrap*. New York: Chapman & Hall.

Emsley, R., liu, H., Dunn, G., Valeri, L., & VanderWeele, T. (2014). Paramed: A command to perform causal mediation analysis using parametric models. *Stata Journal.*

Emsley, R., Dunn, G., & White, I. R. (2010). Mediation and moderation of treatment effects in randomised controlled trials of complex interventions. *Statistical Methods in Medical Research, 19*(3), 237–270.
Fosen J., Ferkingstad, E., Borgan, Ø., & Aalen, O. O. (2006). Dynamic path analysisa new approach to analyzing time dependent covariates. *Lifetime Data Analysis, 12*, 143–167.
Gelfand, L. A., MacKinnon, D. P., De Rubeis, R. J., & Baraldi, A. N. (2016). Mediation analysis with survival outcomes: Accelerated failure time versus proportional hazards models. *Frontiers in Psychology, 7*, 423.
Geneletti, S. (2007). Identifying direct and indirect effects in a non-counterfactual framework. *Journal of the Royal Statistical Society B, 69*, 199–215.
Greenland, S. (2003). Quantifying biases in causal models:classical confounding versus collider-stratification bias. *Epidemiology, 14*, 300–3067.
Greenland, S., & Robins, J. M. (1986). Identifiability, exchangeability, and epidemiological confounding. *International Journal of Epidemiology, 15*, 413–419.
Harris, H. R., Costenbader, K. H., Mu, F., Kvaskoff, M., Malspeis, S., Karlson, E. W., et al. (2016). Endometriosis and the risks of systemic lupus erythematosus and rheumatoid arthritis in the nurses health study ii. *Annals of the Rheumatic Diseases, 75*, 1279–1284.
Hayes, A. F., & Preacher, K. J. (2010). Quantifying and testing indirect effects in simple mediation models when the constituent paths are non linear. *Multivariate Behavioral Research, 45*, 527–660.
Hernán, M. A., & Taubman, S. L. (2008). Does obesity shorten life? The importance of well-defined interventions to answer causal questions. *International Journal of Obesity, 32*(Suppl 3), S8–S14.
Hudgens, M. G., & Halloran, M. E. (2008). Towards causal inference with interference. *Journal of the American Statistical Association, 103*(482), 832–842.
Jackson, J. W., VanderWeele, T. J., Blacker, D., & Schneeweiss, S. (2015). Mediators of first- versus second-generation antipsychotic-related mortality in older adults. *Epidemiology, 26*, 700709.
Jiang, Z., & VanderWeele, T. (2015). When is the difference method conservative for assessing mediation? *American Journal of Epidemiology, 182*(105–108), 28.
Krebs, N. M., Chen, A., Zhu, J., Sun, D., Liao, J., Stennett, A. L., et al. (2016). Comparison of puff volume with cigarettes per day in predicting nicotine uptake among daily smokers. *American Journal of Epidemiology, 184*(48–57), 27.
Kupers, L. K., Xu, X., Jankipersadsing, S. A., Vaez, A., la-Bastide-van Gemert, S., Scholtens, S. et al. (2015). Dna methylation mediates the effect of maternal smoking during pregnancy on birthweight of the offspring. *International Journal of Epidemiology, 4*, 1224–1237 (2015).
Kushner, S. C., Quilty, L. C., Uliaszek, A. A., McBride, C., & Bagby, R. M. (2016). Therapeutic alliance mediates the association between personality and treatment outcome in patients with major depressive disorder. *Journal of Affective Disorders, 201*, 137–144.
Lange, T., & Hansen, J. V. (2011). Direct and indirect effects in a survival context. *Epidemiology, 22*, 575–581.
Lange, T., Vansteelandt, S., & Bekaert, M. (2012). A simple unified approach for estimating natural direct and indirect effects. *American Journal Epidemiology, 176*, 190–195.
Luo, P., & Geng, Z. (2016). Causal mediation analysis for survival outcome with unobserved mediator-outcome confounders. *Computational Statistics and Data Analysis, 93*, 336–347.
MacKinnon, D. P. (2008). *Introduction to statistical mediation analysis*. New York, US: Taylor & Francis.
MacKinnon, D., Lockwood, C. M., Hoffman, J. M., West, S. G., & Sheets, V. (2002). A comparison of methods to test mediation and other intervening variable effects. *Psychological Methods, 7*(1), 83–117.
Martinussen, T., & Vansteelandt, S. (2013). Cox and aalen regression models. *Lifetime Data Analysis, 19*, 279–96.
Martinussen, T., Vansteelandt, S., Gerster, M., & Hjelmborg, J. B. (2011). Estimation of direct effects for survival data by using the Aalen additive hazards model. *Journal of the Royal Statistical Society. Series B, Statistical Methodology, 73*(5), 773–788.

Mendola, P., Mumford, S. L., Mnnisto, T. I., Holston, A., Reddy, U. M., & Laughon, S. K. (2015). Controlled direct effects of preeclampsia on neonatal health after accounting for mediation by preterm bir th epidemiology. *Epidemiology*, *26*, 17–26.

Muthén, B. (2011). *Applications of causally defined direct and indirect effects in mediation analysis using SEM in Mplus*.

Naimi, A. I., Kaufman, J. S., & MacLehose, R. F. (2014). Mediation misgivings: am-biguous clinical and public health interpretations of natural direct and indirect effects. *International Journal of Epidemiology*.

Naimi, A. I., Schnitzer, M. I., Moodie, L. M., & Bodnar, E. E. M. (2016). Mediation analysis for health disparities research. *American Journal of Epidemiology, 184*, 315–324.

Nemes, S., Parris, T. Z., Danielsson, A., Einbeigi, Z., Steineck, G., Jonasson, J. M., et al. (2013). Integrative genomics with mediation analysis in a survival context. *Computational and Mathematical Methods in Medicine*.

Nguyen, Q. C., Osypuk, T. L., Schmidt, N. M., Glymour, M. M., & Tchetgen Tchetgen, E. J. (2015). Practical guidance for conducting mediation analysis with multiple mediators using inverse odds ratio weighting. *American Journal of Epidemiology*.

Nguyen, T. T. X., Tchetgen-Tchetgen, E., Kawachi, I., Gilman, S. E., Walter, S., & Gly- mour, M. (2016). Comparing alternative effect decomposition methods: The role of literacy in mediating educational effects on mortality. *Epidemiology, 27*, 670–676.

Pearce. A., Sawyer, A. C. P., Chittleborough, C. R., Mittinty, M. N., Law, C., & Lynch, J.W. (2016). Do early life cognitive ability and self-regulation skills explain socioeconomic inequalities in academic achievement? an effect decomposition analysis in uk and australian cohorts. *Social Science and Medicine, 165*, 108–118.

Pearl, J. (2001). Direct and indirect effects. In *Proceedings of the Seventeenth Conference on Uncertainty in Artificial Intelligence* (pp. 411–420). San Francisco, CA: Morgan Kaufmann.

Pearl, J. (2010). On the consistency rule in causal inference: Axiom, definition, assumption, or theorem? *Epidemiology*, *21*(6), 872–875.

Petersen, M. L., Sinisi, S. E., & van der Laan, M. J. (2006). Estimation of direct causal effects. *Epidemiology*, *17*(3), 276–284.

Rauscher, G. H., Campbell, R. T., Wiley, E. L., Hoskins, K., Stolley, M. R., & Warnecke, R. B. (2016). Mediation of racial and ethnic disparities in estrogen/progesterone receptornegative breast cancer by socioeconomic position and reproductive factors. *American Journal of Epidemiology, 183*, 884–893.

Richardson, T. S., & Robins, J. (2013). *Single world intervention graphs (swigs): A unification of the counterfactual and graphical approaches to causality*. Technical Report 128, Center for Statistics and the Social Sciences, University of Washington. 30.

Robins, J. (1986). A new approach to causal inference in mortality studies with a sustained exposure period I application to control of the healthy worker survivor effect. *Mathematical Modelling*, *7*(9–12), 1393–1512.

Robins, J. M. (2003). Semantics of causal DAG models and the identification of direct and indirect effects. In P. Green, N. Hjort, & S. Richardson (Eds.), *Highly structured stochastic systems* (pp. 70–81). London: Oxford University Press.

Robins, J. M., & Greenland, S. (1992). Identifiability and exchangeability for direct and indirect effects. *Epidemiology*, *3*(2), 143–155.

Robins, J. M., & Richardson, T. S. (2010). Alternative graphical causal models and the identification of direct effects. In P. Shrout (Ed.), *Causality and psychopathology: Finding the determinants of disorders and their cures* (pp. 103–158). Oxford: Oxford University Press.

Rodgers, S., Vandeleur, C. L., Ajdacic-Gross, V., Aleksandrowicz, A. A., Strippoli M. P. F., Castelao, E. et al. (2016). Tracing the associations between sex, the atypical and the combined atypical-melancholic depression subtypes: A path analysis. *Journal of Affective Disorders, 190*, 807–818.

Rubin, D. B. (1974). Estimating causal effects of treatments in randomized and nonrandomized studies. *Journal of Educational Psychology*, *66*(5), 688–701.

Rubin, D. B. (1980). Comment on: randomization analysis of experimental data: The fisher randomization test. *Journal of the American Statistical Association*, *75*(371), 591–593.

Tchetgen Tchetgen, E. J. (2011). On causal mediation analysis with a survival outcome. *The International Journal of Biostatistics, 7*, 1–38.

Tchetgen Tchetgen, E. (2013). Inverse odds ratio-weighted estimation for causal mediation analysis. *Statistics in Medicine,32*, 4567–4580.

Tchetgen Tchetgen, E. J., & VanderWeele, T. J. (2013). On causal inference in the presence of interference. *Statistical Methods in Medical Research, 21*(1):55–75, 2012.

Tchetgen Tchetgen, E. J., & VanderWeele, T. J. (2014). On identification of natural direct effects when a confounder of the mediator is directly affected by exposure. *Epidemiology, 25*(2), 282–291.

Tein, J.-Y., & MacKinnon, D. P. (2003). Estimating mediated effects with survival data. In H. Yanai, A. Okada, K. Shigemasu, Y. Kano, & J. J. Meulman, (Eds.) *New Developments in Psychometrics: Proceedings of the International Meeting of the Psychometric Society IMPS 2001* (pp. 405–412). Tokyo: Springer. 31.

Tingley, D., Yamamoto, T., Hirose, K., Keele, L., & Imai, K. (2011) Mediation: R package for causal mediation analysis. *Missing*.

Valeri, L., & VanderWeele, T. J. (2013). Mediation analysis allowing for exposure-mediator interactions and causal interpretation: Theoretical assumptions and implementation with sas and spss macros. *Psychological Methods*, *18*, 137–150.

Valeri, L., & VanderWeele, T. J. (2015). Sas macro for causal mediation analysis with survival data. *Epidemiology*, *26*, e23–e24.

van der Laan, M. J., & Rose, S. (2011). *Targeted learning: Causal inference for observational and experimental data*. Springer.

van Iersel, K. C., Kiesner, J., Pastore, M., & Scholte, R. H. J. (2016). The impact of menstrual cycle-related physical symptoms on daily activities and psychological wellness among adolescent girls. *Journal of Adolescence*, *49*, 81–90.

VanderWeele, T. J. (2015). *Explanation in Causal Inference: Methods for Mediation and Interaction*. Oxford University Press.

VanderWeele, T. J. (2009a). Marginal structural models for the estimation of direct and indirect effects. *Epidemiology*, *10*(1), 18–26.

VanderWeele, T. J. (2009b). Mediation and mechanism. *European Journal of Epidemiology*, *24*(5), 217–224.

VanderWeele, T. J. (2009c). Concerning the consistency assumption in causal inference. *Epidemiology*, *20*(6), 880–883.

VanderWeele, T. J. (2011). Causal mediation analysis with survival data. *Epidemiology*, *22*, 582–585.

VanderWeele, T. J. (2012). Structural equation modeling and epidemiologic analysis. *American Journal of Epidemiology*, *176*(7), 608–612.

VanderWeele, T. J. (2013). A three-way decomposition of a total effect into direct, indirect, and interactive effects. *Epidemiology*, *24*(224–32), 29.

VanderWeele, T. J., & Shpitser, I. (2010). Bias formulas for sensitivity analysis for direct and indirect effects. *Epidemiology*, *21*(4), 540–551.

VanderWeele, T., & Vansteelandt, S. (2009). Conceptual issues concerning mediation, interventions and composition. *Statistics and Its Interface*, *2*, 457–468.

VanderWeele, T. J., & Vansteelandt, S. (2010). Odds ratios for mediation analysis for a dichoto-mous outcome. *American Journal of Epidemiology*, *172*(12), 1339–1348.

VanderWeele, T. J., Vansteelandt, S., & Robins, J. M. (2014). Effect decomposition in the presence if an exposure-induced mediator-outcome confounder. *Epidemiology*, *25*(2), 300–306.

Vansteelandt, S. (2012). Estimation of direct and indirect effects. In C. Berzuini, A. P. Dawid, & L. Bernardinelli (Eds.), *Causality: Statistical perspectives and applications* (pp. 126–150). Chichester: Wiley.

Vansteelandt, S., Bekaert, M., & Lange, T. (2012). Imputation strategies for the estimation of natural direct and indirect effects. *Epidemiologic Methods*, *1*, 131–158.

Vansteelandt, S., & Daniel, R. M. (2016). Interventional effects with multiple mediators. *Epidemiology (in press)*, *1*, 1–8.

Vansteelandt, S., & Joffe, M. (2014). Structural nested models and g-estimation: the partially realized promise. *Statistical Science*, *29*(4), 707–731.

Vansteelandt, S., & VanderWeele, T. J. (2012). Natural direct and indirect effects on the exposed: Effect decomposition under weaker assumptions. *Biometrics*, *68*(4), 1019–1027.

Winship, C., & Mare, R. D. (1982). Structural equations and path analysis for discrete data. *American Journal of Sociology*, *88*, 54–110.

Wright, S. (1934). The method of path coeffcients. *Annals of Mathematical Statistics*, *5*, 161–215.

Zhang, Y. T., Laraia, B. A., Mujahid, M. S., Tamayo, A., Blanchard, S. D., Warton, E. M., et al. (2015). Does food vendor density mediate the association between neighborhood deprivation and bmi?: A g-computation mediation analysis. *Epidemiology*, *26*, 344352.

Zheng, W., & van der Laan, M. J. (2012). Targeted maximum likelihood estimation of natural direct effects. *The International Journal of Biostatistics*, *8*, Article 1.

Chapter 2
Lifelong Socio-economic Position and Later Life Health Related Behaviour: A Formal Mediation Approach

George B. Ploubidis, Lenka Benova, Bianca De Stavola and Emily Grundy

Abstract Population ageing is one of the dominant trends of the 21st century. As morbidity and disability are concentrated in the older population, interventions to promote healthy ageing are needed in order to offset the effects that ageing will have on population health. Health related behaviour is a focal area for possible interventions since its association with various health outcomes is well documented. We used data from the English Longitudinal Study of Ageing, with a formal approach for the identification of mediating factors, in order to investigate the lifecourse socio-economic patterning of smoking, physical activity, dietary habits and alcohol use in later life. We found socio-economic gradients in smoking, physical activity and alcohol use, but fewer in healthy dietary habits. Both early and later life socio-economic circumstances influenced health related behaviour, but these associations differed between men and women as well as between age groups. We found that early life circumstances influence behaviour either directly or indirectly 65 years later. The complexity of the observed associations highlights the need for further research on the mechanisms underlying links between socio-economic position and later life health related behaviour.

Keywords Socio-economic position · Health related behaviour · Life course

---

G. B. Ploubidis (✉)
Centre for Longitudinal Studies, UCL Institute of Education, University College London, London, UK
e-mail: G.Ploubidis@UCL.ac.uk

L. Benova
Institute of Tropical Medicine, Antwerp, Belgium
e-mail: lenka.benova@lshtm.ac.uk

B. De Stavola
GOS Institute of Child Health, University College London, London, UK
e-mail: b.destavola@ucl.ac.uk

E. Grundy
Institute for Social and Economic Research, University of Essex, Colchester, UK
e-mail: emily.grundy@essex.ac.uk

G. B. Ploubidis et al., *Pathways to Health*,
SpringerBriefs in Population Studies,
https://doi.org/10.1007/978-94-024-1707-4_2

2.1 Introduction

Population ageing is one of the dominant trends of the 21st century and presents a challenge for the future sustainability of pension and health care systems. As morbidity is concentrated in the older population, interventions outside the medical system to promote healthy ageing are needed in order to offset the effects that ageing will have on population health. Health related lifestyles, including behaviours such as smoking, physical activity, dietary habits and alcohol use are a focal area for possible interventions since the association between these behaviours and various health outcomes is well documented (Birnie et al., 2011; Doll, Peto, Boreham, & Sutherland, 2004; Kannel & Sorlie, 1979; Leon, Saburova, Tomkins, McKee, & Shkolnikov, 2007; Warburton, Nicol, & Bredin, 2006).

Consequently health-related behaviour has been cited alongside educational opportunities, income distribution and access to healthcare as an important domain in which interventions may improve health outcomes (Mackenbach et al., 2008). It has also been argued that advanced welfare states have now reached the fourth stage of the epidemiological transition in which health improvement depends to a large extent on behaviour change (Mackenbach, 2012). It is well recognised that differences in health and in mortality by indicators of Socio-Economic Position (SEP) persist at older ages in many contexts, although relative differentials appear lower than in younger age groups (Demakakos, Nazroo, Breeze, & Marmot, 2008; Gjonca, Tabassum, & Breeze, 2009; Grundy & Sloggett, 2003; Huisman, Kunst, & Mackenbach, 2003; Ploubidis, DeStavola, & Grundy, 2011; Ploubidis, Benova, Grundy, Laydon, & DeStavola, 2014; Ploubidis & Grundy, 2009). Changing health related behaviour has the potential to reduce the social gradient in later life health as it lies on one of the pathways that link Socio-Economic Position (SEP) and health (Kaplan, Pamuk, Lynch, Cohen, & Balfour, 1996; Lynch, Smith, Kaplan, & House, 2000; Schrijvers, Stronks, van de Mheen, & Mackenbach, 1999).

These observations suggest that policies targeting health related behaviour have great potential to shift the overall distribution of risk and improve population health (Rose, 1985) For these policies to succeed further understanding of the determinants of later life health related behaviour is needed. In the present study we focus on the association between life-course SEP and later life health related behaviour. Our major aim is to compare the degree of socio-economic patterning of smoking, physical activity, dietary habits and alcohol use in later life and investigate to what extent this is due to early life and/or later life socio-economic circumstances.

2.2 Methods

2.2.1 Sample

We used data from the fourth wave (2009) and the life course interview (third wave—2007) of the English Longitudinal Study of Ageing (ELSA), a nationally representative multi-purpose sample of the population aged 50 and over living in England. The ELSA sample was drawn from households that responded to the 1998, 1999 or 2001 rounds of the Health Survey for England (HSE), a stratified random sample of all households in England. Response rates to these HSE rounds were 69%, 70% and 67% respectively (Marmot, Banks, Blundell, Lessof, & Nazroo, 2002). A comparison of the socio-demographic characteristics of the ELSA with national census data indicated that the ELSA sample was representative of the non-institutionalised population (Marmot et al., 2002). Our analytic sample included participants with at least one valid observation on the early life SEP indicators measured in the ELSA Wave 3 life-course interview (N = 7578, out of 7855 eligible participants). From the participants that took part on the ELSA life-course interview at Wave 3, some information was lost due to attrition on Wave 4 (74% of participants in Wave 3 participated in Wave 4). Consequently in the variables measured at Wave 4, valid information was available for 6683 participants. Preliminary results (not shown here) confirmed that the distribution of demographic characteristics such as gender and marital status, as well as self-rated health status of the participants in our analytic sample was similar to national census data, indicating that it remains broadly representative of the non-institutionalised older population of England.

2.2.2 Measures

Recollection of early life SEP and health—ELSA Life history interview (Wave 3—2007)
We combined several indicators of participants' recall of early life SEP (at age 10) and early life health (childhood and early adolescence) in latent summaries that capture the common variance between these indicators. Paternal occupational social class, housing tenure, access to household amenities, the number of books in the household and number of persons per room (crowding) were used as indicators of early life SEP. Childhood health status measures were based on self-reported health at age 10; whether participants reported missing school for more than one month; restriction of physical activities for more than 3 months; whether participants recalled being confined to bed for more than one month and whether or not they reported more than three inpatient stays in any one year. Combining several indicators in a latent variable controls for random error which may be present in the recalled indicators of early life SEP and health since participants' childhood was at least four decades in the past (Rabe-Hesketh & Skrondal, 2008). It is recognised that current health

status may influence recall of health of health in the past. In order to control for such concurrent to recall health status (presence of chronic illness and depression at the time of recall—both measured at ELSA Wave 3) we used a Multiple Indicators Multiple Causes (MIMIC) model in order to capture the influence of systematic recall bias. We note that the questions on early life circumstances, depression and presence of chronic illness were asked at Wave 3 (2007), whereas both our health outcomes are derived from ELSA wave 4 which took place two years later (2009). High scores in the latent summaries represent high SEP and optimal health (see Electronic Supplementary Material—I, for frequency distribution of all early life indicators).

Later life measures—ELSA Wave 4 (2009)
We employed a latent summary of later life SEP based on net individual income and total net wealth using the approach described in Ploubidis, DeStavola and Grundy (2011), with high scores representing high SEP. We employed a binary self-reported measure of current smoking status, and three binary outcomes representing whether participants engaged in mild, moderate and/or vigorous physical activity more than once a week. We derived a latent summary measure of alcohol use, combining information from five self-reported questions: whether the respondent had an alcoholic drink last week, how many drinks the respondent had last week and the number of units of spirits, glasses of wine and pints of beer consumed during the last week. A high score on the alcohol summary measure indicates high alcohol use. Similarly we derived a latent summary measure of healthy dietary habits combining items that enquired about the amount of fruit and vegetables the participants consumed last month and last week. High scores on the healthy diet summary indicate frequent consumption of fruit and vegetables.

Confounders
Age, gender, marital status, employment status, number of children, presence of chronic illness and cognitive ability were included in the model as they are thought to be important confounders of the association between the main mediator of interest, later life SEP, and the six health related behaviour outcomes.

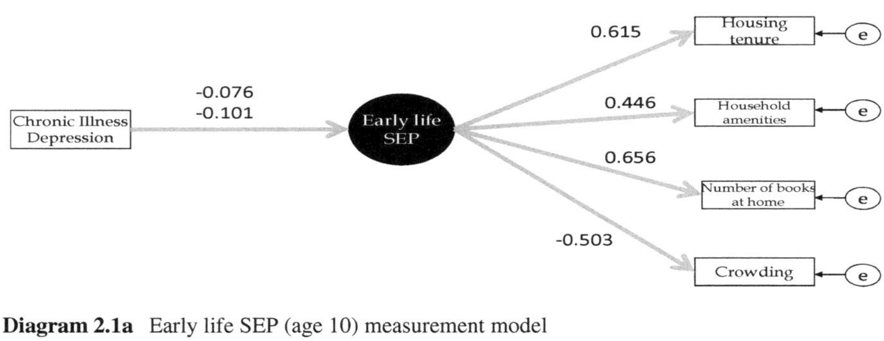

Diagram 2.1a Early life SEP (age 10) measurement model

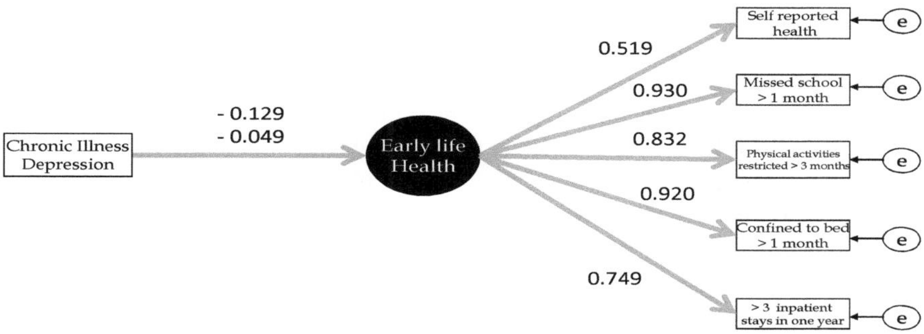

Diagram 2.1b Early life health (childhood and early adolescence) measurement model

2.2.3 *Statistical Modelling*

In order to formally compare the relative contribution of early life and later life SEP on health related behaviour, direct and indirect effects and their standard errors need to be appropriately quantified. In the causal mediation literature several approaches have been proposed for the estimation of direct and indirect effects with an emphasis on different aspects of mediation (Snowden, Rose, & Mortimer, 2011; Ten Have & Joffe, 2012; Vanderweele, 2012; Daniel, De Stavola, & Cousens, 2011).

In the case of alcohol use and diet scores, all variables of interest were continuous and approximately normally distributed. Mediation within linear systems can be reliably quantified with Linear Structural Equation Models (De Stavola, Daniel, Ploubidis, & Micali, 2015; Ten Have & Joffe, 2012). Therefore for both these outcomes LSEM models were estimated with the robust maximum likelihood (MLR) estimator in Mplus 6.1 [18] and all reported model parameters are standardized so that their relative sizes can be compared. It has been shown that in the presence of binary or ordinal mediators and/or outcomes causal mediation approaches are needed in order to appropriately quantify the direct and indirect effects (Imai, Keele, & Tingley, 2010; Ten Have & Joffe, 2012). In order to appropriately quantify the direct and indirect effects of SEP on the four binary outcomes (smoking, mild, moderate and vigorous physical activity), we employed the G formula which has been shown to produce reliable estimates in such scenarios (Daniel et al., 2011). We report the Randomised Interventional Analogue of the Natural Indirect Effects (Vanderweele, Vansteelandt, & Robins, 2014) as reported in Chap. 1 of this volume.

Considering that unbiased estimates of pathways cannot be obtained without properly addressing the implications of incompleteness of data we employed the Full Information Maximum Likelihood method which is naturally incorporated into LSEM. In this approach the selection mechanism is ignorable under the Missing at Random (MAR) assumption (Little & Rubin, 1989, 2002). In this case MAR implies that the if all the variables that are responsible for the missing data generating mechanism are included in the model, then this can be ignored and parameter estimates can be robustly computed for participants with missing data. Practically, in our analysis

MAR translates to the following assumption: all systematic missingness is due to variables included in our models, the exposure (early life SEP), mediators (early life health and later life SEP) and mediator—outcome confounders (later life cognitive ability, age, marital status and employment status). Any other missingness that is not accounted for by these variables is thought to be random (thus missing at random, since we assume that all systematic causes of attrition have been included in the model). We believe that this is a reasonable assumption since it has been shown that SEP and age are the main drivers of attrition in population surveys in the UK (Durrant & Goldstein, 2008), as well as in the ELSA (Steptoe, Breeze, Banks, & Nazroo, 2012).

2.3 Results

Table 2.1 shows descriptive statistics for the exposure (early life SEP), mediators (early life Health and later life SEP) and outcomes (current smoking status, mild, moderate and vigorous physical activity, alcohol use and consumption of fruit and vegetables) in the model. In Tables 2.2 and 2.3 and Figs. 2.1, 2.2, 2.3, 2.4, 2.5 and 2.6 we present the odds ratios and standardised parameters where appropriate and 95% confidence intervals for the six groups (Diagram 2.1a).

Measurement models for recollection of early life SEP and health

In Diagram 2.1a we present the standardised factor loadings of all early life SEP indicators that can be interpreted as correlations between the indicators and the latent variable. All loadings were satisfactory > |0.4|, but none exceeded |0.662|, indicating the presence of random error in all early life SEP indicators that was excluded from valid early life SEP variance which is represented by the latent variable. With respect to systematic error in the form of recall bias due to concurrent to the time of recall chronic illness and depression, the presence of one or more chronic illnesses was negatively associated with early life SEP, b = −0.076 (−0.107 to −0.044) as was depression b = −0.101 (−0.134 to −0.069). In Graph 3 we present the standardised factor loadings of all early life health indicators. All standardised loadings were satisfactory > |0.74|, with the exception of self-rated health during childhood, which was the only early life health item affected substantively by random error. The presence of one or more chronic illnesses at the time of recall was negatively associated with recollections of early life health, b = −0.129 (−0.160 to −0.098), as was depression b = −0.049 (−0.079 to −0.019) (Diagram 2.1b).

Smoking

In men later life SEP was negatively associated with smoking in all age groups indicating that those with more advantaged SEP tend not to smoke. Early life SEP was only indirectly (via later life SEP) related with smoking in those under 75. In women under 75 both early life and later life SEP were negatively associated with smoking. Early life SEP had both direct and indirect—via later life SEP—effects on smoking. However, neither early life nor later life SEP were associated with smoking

Table 2.1 Descriptive statistics of exposures, mediators and outcomes in the model

		Men			Women		
Continuous variables	Age group	N	Mean	Std. deviation	N	Mean	Std. deviation
Early life SEP at age 10	50–64	1738	0.35	0.75	2143	0.43	0.75
Wave 3	65–74	920	0.11	0.78	1084	0.21	0.85
	75+	702	−0.04	0.78	971	0.02	0.84
	Total	3360	0.20	0.78	4198	0.28	0.82
Early life health	50–64	1738	1.26	0.76	2143	1.33	0.74
Wave 3	65–74	919	1.21	0.77	1082	1.13	0.79
	75+	702	1.20	0.73	969	1.16	0.78
	Total	3359	1.24	0.76	4194	1.24	0.77
Later life SEP	50–64	1556	0.15	0.79	1911	0.05	0.82
Wave 4	65–74	823	0.05	0.75	991	−0.06	0.74
	75+	584	−0.05	0.71	814	−0.32	0.66
	Total	2963	0.08	0.77	3716	−0.06	0.78
Alcohol use score	50–64	1359	0.24	0.84	1703	−0.12	0.87
Wave 4	65–74	745	0.25	0.91	885	−0.23	0.96
	75+	459	0.05	1.06	646	−0.37	1.01
	Total	2563	0.21	0.91	3234	−0.20	0.93
Healthy diet score	50–64	1362	−0.02	0.76	1706	−0.01	0.74
Wave 4	65–74	740	0.04	0.80	896	0.01	0.69
	75+	456	0.02	0.76	658	0.08	0.77
	Total	2558	0.00	0.77	3260	0.01	0.73
		Men			Women		
Binary variables	Age group	N	%		N	%	
Currently smokes	50–64	1547	15.7		1903	17.8	
Wave 4	65–74	817	13.0		977	10.1	
	75+	575	4.9		811	7.0	
	Total	2939	12.8		3691	13.4	

(continued)

Table 2.1 (continued)

		Men			Women		
Binary variables	Age group	N	%		N	%	
Mild physical activity > once a week	50–64	1551	86.7		1911	94.5	
Wave 4	65–74	820	83.5		987	91.0	
			74.1		825	75.6	
	Total	2958	83.3		3723	89.4	
Moderate physical activity > once a week	50–64	1551	85.5		1910	81.6	
Wave 4	65–74	820	80.4		987	72.2	
	75+	587	63.4		825	43.9	
	Total	2958	79.7		3722	70.7	
Vigorous physical activity > once a week	50–64	1551	39.6		1910	32.0	
Wave 4	65–74	820	33.2		987	25.5	
	75+	587	18.1		825	8.4	
	Total	2958	33.5		3722	25.1	

in women over 75. In both men and women early life health was not associated with smoking in later life, possibly because of selection due to differential mortality.

Mild physical activity
In men only later life SEP was associated with mild physical activity, with high SEP increasing the probability of mild physical activity. Early life SEP was only indirectly associated with mild physical activity. In women later life SEP was also positively associated with mild physical activity while—as in men—early life SEP influenced later life mild physical activity indirectly via later life SEP. Early life health was not associated with mild physical activity.

Moderate physical activity
Later life SEP was positively associated with moderate physical activity in men of all age groups. Furthermore, later life SEP fully mediated the effect of early life SEP on moderate physical activity. In women both early and later life SEP were positively associated with moderate physical activity. Early SEP was directly associated with

Table 2.2 Standardised parameters and 95% confidence intervals—men

Age group	Smoking	Mild PA	Moderate PA	Vigorous PA	Alcohol	Diet
50–64						
Later life SEP	**0.576 (0.488 to 0.681)**	**1.453 (1.217 to 1.735)**	**1.509 (1.279 to 1.780)**	**1.362 (1.204 to 1.542)**	**0.152 (0.092 to 0.212)**	**0.085 (0.024 to 0.145)**
Early life SEP	1.012 (0.870 to 1.177)	1.091 (0.923 to 1.288)	1.017 (0.874 to 1.184)	1.082 (0.963 to 1.214)	**0.063 (0.007 to 0.119)**	0.023 (−0.035 to 0.081)
Early life SEP via later Life SEP	**0.509 (0.392 to 0.663)**	**1.476 (1.158 to 1.896)**	**1.599 (1.282 to 1.995)**	**1.379 (1.187 to 1.604)**	**0.049 (0.029 to 0.070)**	0.007 (−0.012 to 0.026)
Total early life SEP	0.537 (0.259 to 1.126)	2.310 (0.984 to 5.528)	1.845 (0.863 to 3.951)	**1.934 (1.212 to 3.089)**	**0.112 (0.057 to 0.168)**	0.050 (−0.007 to 0.107)
Early life health	0.972 (0.839 to1.128)	1.037 (0.896 to 1.201)	**1.173 (1.006 to 1.368)**	1.089 (0.978 to 1.212)	0.035 (−0.015 to 0.085)	0.012 (−0.040 to 0.063)
65–74						
Later life SEP	**0.496 (0.377 to 0.653)**	1.222 (0.971 to 1.538)	**1.841 (1.463 to 2.318)**	**1.398 (1.174 to 1.665)**	**0.233 (0.155 to 0.311)**	0.009 (−0.074 to 0.091)
Early life SEP	0.969 (0.739 to 1.271)	1.217 (0.968 to 1.529)	1.058 (0.856 to 1.308)	1.003 (0.853 to 1.180)	**0.084 (0.010 to 0.158)**	0.039 (−0.043 to 0.122)
Early life SEP via later Life SEP	**0.537 (0.367 to 0.786)**	1.196 (0.879 to 1.627)	**2.009 (1.447 to 2.787)**	**1.404 (1.099 to 1.794)**	**0.090 (0.056 to 0.124)**	0.003 (−0.028 to 0.035)
Total early life SEP	0.491 (0.177 to 1.363)	**2.801 (1.015 to 7.729)**	**2.756 (1.145 to 6.619)**	1.471 (0.774 to 2.784)	**0.174 (0.103 to 0.245)**	0.043 (−0.036 to 0.121)
Early life health	1.024 (0.831 to 1.262)	0.941 (0.787 to 1.124)	1.125 (0.938 to 1.350)	0.910 (0.780 to 1.061)	0.050 (−0.024 to 0.124)	0.058 (−0.015 to 0.130)
75+						
Later life SEP	**0.571 (0.327 to 0.997)**	**1.849 (1.446 to 2.363)**	**1.605 (1.284 to 2.007)**	1.226 (0.926 to 1.622)	**0.186 (0.083 to 0.290)**	0.063 (−0.059 to 0.185)
Early life SEP	0.973 (0.641 to 1.478)	0.884 (0.71 to 71.09)	0.882 (0.720 to 1.081)	0.861 (0.671 to 1.105)	**0.116 (0.019 to 0.214)**	−0.082 (−0.179 to 0.014)
Early life SEP via later life SEP	0.778 (0.554 to 1.094)	**2.164 (1.520 to 3.080)**	**1.928 (1.439 to 2.585)**	1.160 (0.423 to 1.466)	**0.074 (0.031 to 0.118)**	0.025 (−0.024 to 0.074)
Total early life SEP	0.670 (0.244 to 1.840)	1.335 (0.644 to 2.767)	1.268 (0.618 to 2.609)	0.788 (0.405 to 1.529)	**0.191 (0.099 to 0.283)**	−0.057 (−0.158 to 0.043)
Early life health	1.163 (0.773 to 1.749)	0.933 (0.764 to 1.139)	**0.814 (0.663 to 0.999)**	0.891 (0.721 to 1.099)	0.017 (−0.068 to 0.102)	0.020 (−0.070 to 0.110)

PA physical activity

[a]Parameters adjusted for age, marital status, employment status, number of children and cognitive ability (all confounders from ELSA Wave 4)

Table 2.3 Standardised parameters and 95% confidence intervals—women

Age group	Smoking	Mild PA	Moderate PA	Vigorous PA	Alcohol	Diet
50–64						
Later life SEP	**0.609 (0.526 to 0.706)**	1.275 (0.998 to 1.629)	**1.449 (1.255 to 1.673)**	**1.586 (1.407 to 1.787)**	**0.277 (0.225 to 0.328)**	**0.122 (0.067 to 0.177)**
Early life SEP	**0.831 (0.727 to 0.949)**	1.168 (0.943 to 1.446)	**1.199 (1.053 to 1.364)**	**1.232 (1.105 to 1.374)**	**0.079 (0.029 to 0.129)**	**0.100 (0.049 to 0.152)**
Early life SEP via later life SEP	**0.561 (0.446 to 0.704)**	**1.429 (1.001 to 2.033)**	**1.606 (1.284 to 2.011)**	**1.710 (1.370 to 2.138)**	**0.091 (0.070 to 0.111)**	**0.033 (0.015 to 0.050)**
Total early life SEP	**0.219 (0.115 to 0.415)**	**3.296 (1.049 to 6.277)**	**4.075 (2.205 to 7.538)**	**5.424 (2.559 to 11.484)**	**0.170 (0.121 to 0.219)**	**0.133 (0.090 to 0.191)**
Early life health	1.029 (0.909 to 1.166)	1.091 (0.884 to 1.348)	**1.140 (1.015 to 1.279)**	1.047 (0.939 to 1.169)	0.028 (−0.016 to 0.072)	0.006 (−0.041 to 0.053)
65–74						
Later life SEP	**0.623 (0.468 to 0.831)**	**1.398 (1.174 to 1.665)**	**1.469 (1.219 to 1.769)**	1.176 (0.997 to 1.387)	**0.275 (0.201 to 0.348)**	0.046 (−0.028 to 0.119)
Early life SEP	**0.707 (0.549 to 0.909)**	1.003 (0.853 to 1.180)	1.124 (0.958 to 1.319)	1.061 (0.899 to 1.251)	**0.150 (0.081 to 0.219)**	**0.086 (0.012 to 0.160)**
Early life SEP via later life SEP	**0.477 (0.304 to 0.742)**	1.523 (0.974 to 1.090)	**1.678 (1.275 to 2.210)**	1.191 (0.928 to 1.529)	**0.099 (0.068 to 0.130)**	0.017 (−0.010 to 0.043)
Total early life SEP	**0.098 (0.035 to 0.275)**	1.629 (0.590 to 4.504)	**2.756 (1.443 to 5.264)**	1.469 (0.758 to 2.849)	**0.249 (0.184 to 0.313)**	**0.103 (0.033 to 0.172)**
Early life health	0.937 (0.747 to 1.176)	0.910 (0.780 to 1.061)	1.026 (0.883 to 1.192)	1.051 (0.907 to 1.218)	0.049 (−0.011 to 0.108)	−0.013 (−0.077 to 0.052)
75+						
Later life SEP	0.889 (0.674 to 1.173)	**1.369 (1.131 to 1.656)**	**1.241 (1.055 to 1.460)**	1.261 (0.976 to 1.630)	**0.235 (0.152 to 0.318)**	0.001 (−0.086 to 0.088)
Early life SEP	0.899 (0.696 to 1.163)	1.121 (0.680 to 1.533)	**1.198 (1.019 to 1.409)**	1.145 (0.870 to 1.507)	**0.164 (0.079 to 0.248)**	**0.085 (0.005 to 0.165)**
Early life SEP via later life SEP	0.886 (0.659 to 1.191)	**1.237 (1.013 to 1.509)**	**1.171 (1.001 to 1.371)**	1.080 (0.847 to 1.377)	**0.057 (0.032 to 0.082)**	0.001 (−0.021 to 0.021)
Total early life SEP	0.612 (0.169 to 2.212)	2.083 (0.967 to 4.490)	**2.073 (1.053 to 4.075)**	1.248 (0.409 to 3.807)	**0.221 (0.134 to 0.307)**	**0.085 (0.006 to 0.164)**
Early life health	0.781 (1.048 to 1.407)	1.045 (0.869 to 1.257)	**1.191 (1.022 to 1.388)**	1.180 (0.898 to 1.550)	−0.046 (−0.118 to 0.027)	0.029 (−0.048 to 0.105)

PA physical activity

[a]Parameters adjusted for age, marital status, employment status, number of children and cognitive ability (all confounders from ELSA Wave 4)

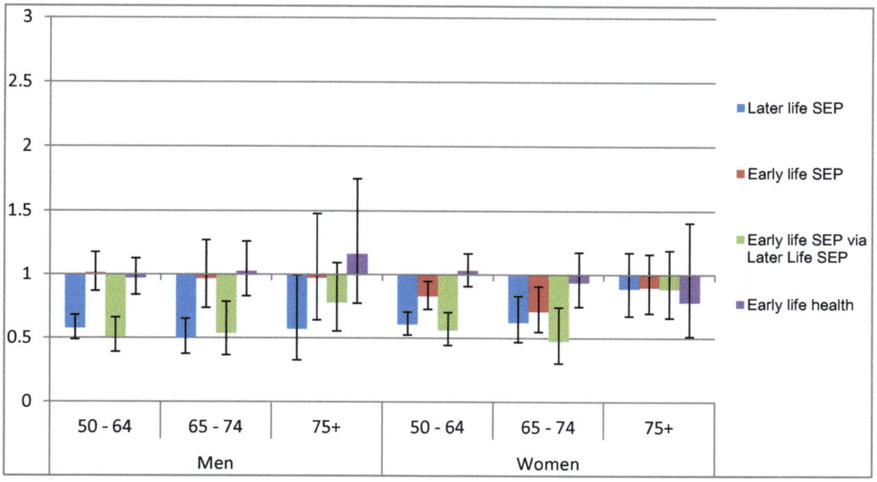

Fig. 2.1 Odds ratios and 95% confidence intervals—current smoking

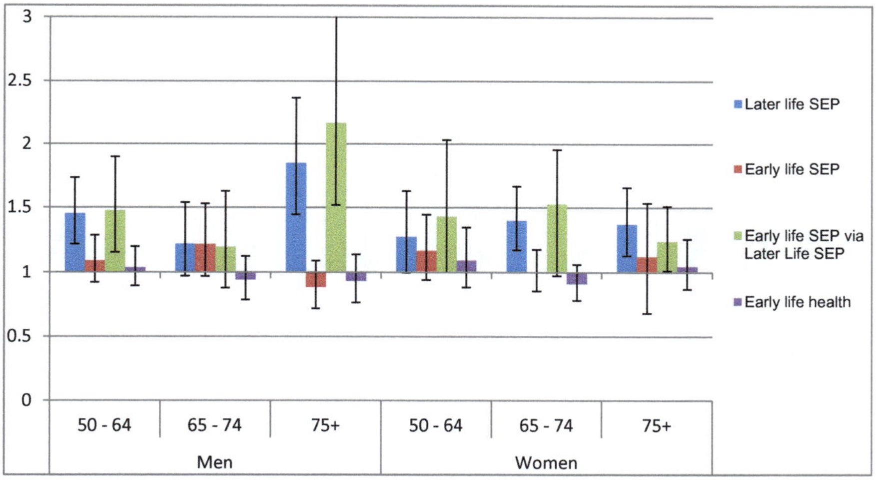

Fig. 2.2 Odds ratios and 95% confidence intervals—mild physical activity

moderate physical activity with an effect of a similar magnitude to that of life SEP. The total effect of early life SEP (direct plus indirect via later life SEP) was stronger compared to the effect of later life SEP. Men and women with good early life health were more likely to engage to moderate physical activity in later life, and the effect was observed in both those under 65 and over 75.

Vigorous physical activity

In men only later life SEP was associated with engaging in vigorous physical activity more than once a week, and the association was observed only for those under 75.

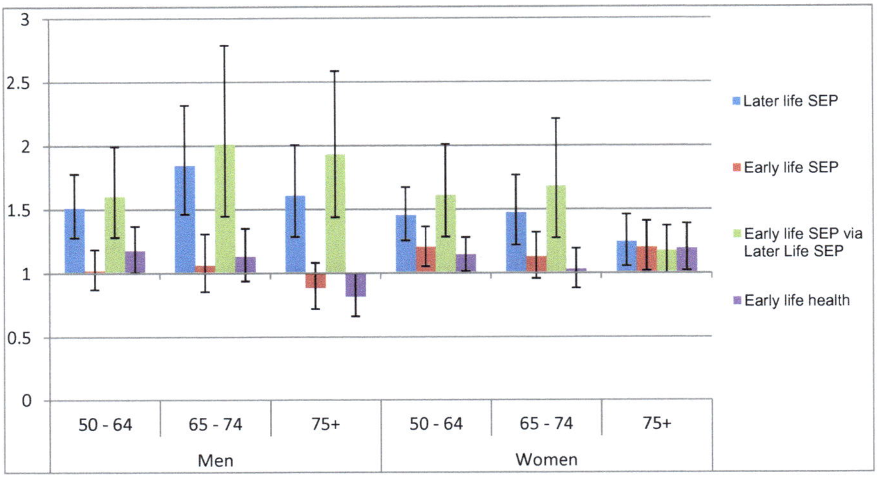

Fig. 2.3 Odds ratios and 95% confidence intervals—moderate physical activity

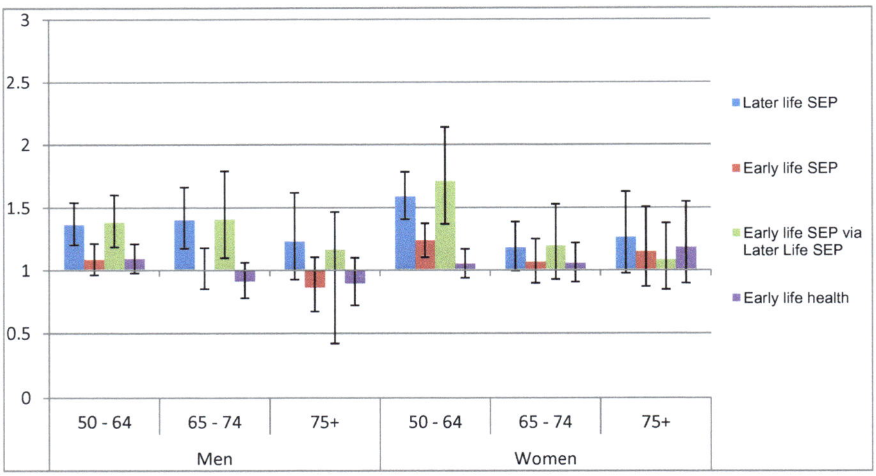

Fig. 2.4 Odds ratios and 95% confidence intervals—vigorous physical activity

In women under 65 both early life and later life SEP were associated with vigorous physical activity. We did not observe an effect of early or later life SEP for women over 65.

Alcohol use
Early life and later life SEP were both positively associated with alcohol use. The effects were observed in both genders, although in women the effect was stronger,

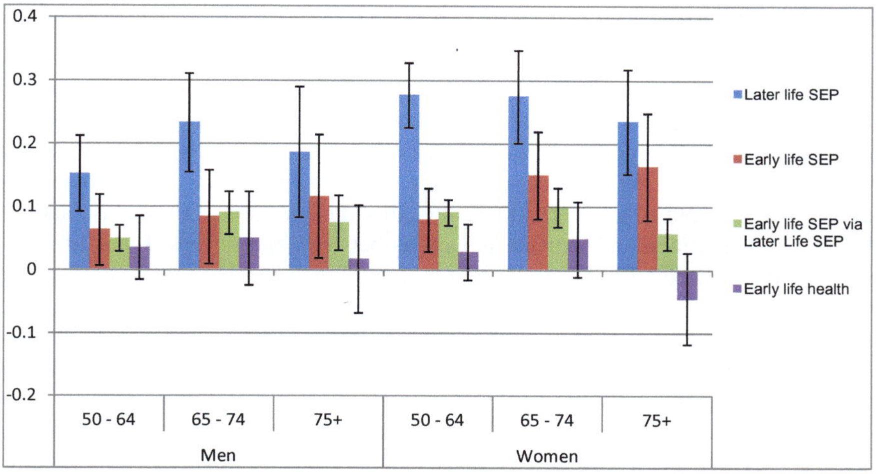

Fig. 2.5 Standardised parameters and 95% confidence intervals—alcohol use score

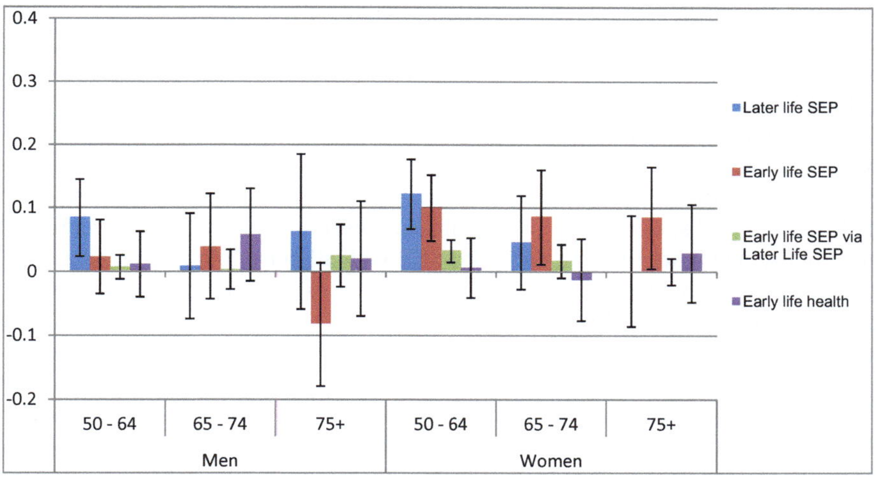

Fig. 2.6 Standardised parameters and 95% confidence intervals—healthy diet score

and in all age groups. The effect of early life SEP was more prominent in women. Early life health was not associated with alcohol use.

Diet

Later life SEP was positively associated with the healthy diet score, but only in men and women under 65 years old. Later life SEP was not associated with the healthy diet score in any other age group in both men and women. On the contrary, early life SEP was directly associated with the healthy diet score in women over 65.

2.4 Discussion

The associations between SEP and health related behaviour in early adulthood and midlife are well established. Our results extend this literature by considering associations in later life (Harper et al., 2002; Lynch, Kaplan, & Salonen, 1997; Wardle & Steptoe, 2003). We observed socio-economic gradients in smoking, physical activity and alcohol use, but to a lesser extent in healthy dietary habits. These associations differed between men and women as well as between age groups. Later life SEP dominated the association in smoking in men in all age groups, whereas in women both early life and later life SEP were negatively associated with smoking in those under 75. A homogeneous pattern emerged for all types of physical activity in men, where later life SEP was positively associated with mild, moderate and vigorous physical activity and early life SEP had only an indirect association with all types of activity. A different pattern of associations was observed in women. Only later life SEP was associated with mild physical activity in women over 65, whereas both early and later life SEP were associated with moderate and vigorous physical activity. The associations with SEP were observed in all age groups with the exception of smoking in women and vigorous activity in both genders, where a socio-economic gradient was not observed for men and women over 75. This finding is possibly due to selection effects, since participants with lower SEP that were likely to engage to unhealthy behaviour did not reach that age due to selective mortality.

We found that early life circumstances influence behaviour either directly or indirectly even 65 years later. This finding extends the previously reported associations between early life SEP and midlife health related behaviour (Lynch et al., 1997; van de Mheen, Stronks, Looman, & Mackenbach, 1998). In men, with the exception of alcohol use, the association of early life SEP with all behaviours was mediated by later life SEP, whereas in women direct associations of early life SEP with smoking, moderate and vigorous physical activity, as well as alcohol use and dietary habits were observed. One explanation of these findings comes from the idea of reproduction of social capital. According to Bourdieu (1986) tastes for food and a whole range of lifestyle factors are symbolic of a particular class position. The observation that physical activity, diet, smoking and alcohol use were directly related to early life SEP may reflect the age prior to later life at which particular behaviours became established in the habitual repertoires of the participants of ELSA. Thus, behaviours shared by those with similar SEP at earlier stages of the lifecourse had an independent of later SEP association with later life health behaviour. Previous work investigating the association between early life physical activity and activity on midlife support this theory (Kuh & Cooper, 1992; Tammelin, Nayha, Hills, & Jarvelin, 2003).

The strong associations between SEP at various stages of the life course with all health related behaviours can be explained by characteristics of the physical environment (for example, places to walk, availability of healthy foods), social norms (smoking levels, physical activity and eating habits in the community), and the costs of health protective behaviours. Individual knowledge, attitudinal, and motivational factors stemming from educational access, life experiences, and the general level of health consciousness expressed within the local social environment have also been shown to influence health related behaviour (Harper et al., 2002; Wardle & Steptoe, 2003). Another potential explanation is the possibility that greater fatalism over the future which can influence health behaviour is more prevalent in lower socioeconomic groups. Although this argument has been contested, in ELSA participants' forecasts of how many more years they expected to live were associated with smoking, and diagnoses of cancer and diabetes (Kobayashi, Beeken, & Meisel, 2017). Considering that smoking and being diagnosed with diabetes or cancer are socio-economically patterned (Stringhini, Zaninotto, Kumari, Kivimäki, & Batty, 2016) indicates that at least in the older population less advantaged SEP is associated with more negative expectations about future health status.

Strengths of the present study include the availability of a population based dataset and the formal model based approach in the parameterisation of the effect of lifelong SEP on later life health related behaviour. However, there are some limitations that need to be considered while interpreting our results. First, the problem of unmeasured confounding has yet to be resolved in observational settings and it has been argued that some kind of sensitivity analysis should always be presented when observational data is used (Greenland, 1996). According to the sequential ignorability assumption if unmeasured confounders are suspected our estimated parameters will be biased. For example, parental characteristics, such as cognitive ability and health status were not taken into account in our model (information on these variables is not available in the ELSA) and may have introduced bias in our estimates (Jivraj, Goodman, Ploubidis, & de Oliveira, 2017). We have shown similarities comparing the ELSA with prospectively collected data from the 1958 British birth cohort in the direction and statistical significance of associations, but not in the magnitude of regression coefficients, with the magnitude of the point estimates differing substantially due to the fact that variables such as early life cognitive ability is not available in the ELSA, as it cannot be assessed retrospectively. However, the inclusion of various mediator—outcome confounders, including later life cognitive ability has the potential to "block"—at least partly—the pathways through which unmeasured confounders could bias our results. We note that adjusting for mediator—outcome cofounders that are affected by SEP gives rise to the well-known issue of intermediate confounding (De Stavola et al., 2015). In this instance our findings are valid under the assumption of no interaction between early life SEP, later life SEP and any of the mediator—outcome confounders.

We attempted to quantify these effects by simulating a series of sensitivity analyses where a continuous latent variable was added in the models in order to represent unmeasured parental characteristics. Our observed results remained valid even in strong confounding scenarios, indicating that unmeasured parental characteristics do not account for our results. We have adjusted for potential confounders of the later life SEP and health (mediator—outcome) association and the assumption of no unmeasured mediator—outcome confounders is, we believe, sufficiently approximated. Despite this, we also simulated the effect of potential unmeasured confounders on this association. Our results were supported even under strong mediator—outcome confounding conditions. However, despite our efforts, bias due to unmeasured or residual confounding cannot be ruled out.

Another limitation that should be considered while interpreting our results is that our study relied on self-reported data and It is well known that data from self-reported measures are likely to be biased by some process that is driven by the respondent's personality and circumstances (Groot, 2000; Lindeboom & van Doorslaer, 2004). In the latent summaries in our models (early life SEP and health, later life SEP, alcohol use and dietary habits) self-reporting bias was to a certain accounted for since latent variables capture the common variance between indicators. In practice this means that in order for our summaries to be biased participants would have to give biased responses in all indicators of a summary. However unlikely, we do not know to which extend this misreporting may have occurred. With respect to the observed binary outcomes, such approach is not possible, but all outcomes (binary and continuous) correlate highly and in the expected direction with external objectively measured criteria such the Body Mass Index, Waist—Hip Ratio, timed chair rise stands, grip strength and respiratory function (results available from corresponding author). Another potential source of bias is the retrospective nature of the early life data. However in a previous study using the same data, we have found that systematic bias on recall of early life SEP and health accounted for about 3–7% of the overall valid—excluding random error—variance of both constructs, indicating that responses to questions in the ELSA life course interview are to a large extend driven by correct recall (Ploubidis et al., 2014). Recent work comparing the ELSA and the 1958 British birth cohort show a degree of comparability in salient life events, such as parental separation and being in institutional care in childhood as well as less salient circumstances, such as father's occupation further reinforcing our interpretation that measurement error due to recall bias did not influence our findings (Jivraj et al., 2017).

Despite these limitations, our results extend previous findings on mid adulthood and early old age, to old age and the beginnings of late old age. The complexity of the observed associations which has not been captured by previous research highlights the need for further work on the mechanism that underlies the links between SEP and later life health related behaviour, especially since most of the empirical evidence for explanations of the SEP health behaviour association is derived by studies in midlife. Future studies are needed in order to investigate whether these explanations are relevant for the older population as well as their relative importance in explaining later life health related behaviour, in order to identify meaningful target areas for health related policy.

References

Birnie, K., Ben-Shlomo, Y., Gunnell, D., Ebrahim, S., Bayer, A., Gallacher, J., & Martin, R. M. (2011). Diet in childhood and adulthood and physical performance in old age: Findings from the Boyd Orr and Caerphilly cohorts. *Journal of Epidemiology and Community Health, 65*. https://doi.org/10.1136/jech.2011.143586.77.

Bourdieu, P. (1986). The forms of capital. In J. G. Richardson (Ed.), *Handbook of theory and research for the sociology of education* (pp. 241–258). New York: Greenwood Press.

Daniel, R. M., De Stavola, B. L., & Cousens, S. N. (2011). gformula: Estimating causal effects in the presence of time-varying confounding or mediation using the g-computation formula. *Stata Journal, 11*(4), 479–517.

De Stavola, B. L., Daniel, R. M., Ploubidis, G. B., & Micali, N. (2015). Mediation analysis with intermediate confounding: Structural equation modeling viewed through the causal inference lens. *American Journal of Epidemiology, 181*(1), 64–80. https://doi.org/10.1093/aje/kwu239.

Demakakos, P., Nazroo, J., Breeze, E., & Marmot, M. (2008). Socioeconomic status and health: The role of subjective social status. *Social Science & Medicine, 67*(2), 330–340. https://doi.org/10.1016/j.socscimed.2008.03.038.

Doll, R., Peto, R., Boreham, J., & Sutherland, I. (2004). Mortality in relation to smoking: 50 years' observations on male British doctors. *British Medical Journal, 328*(7455), 1519–1528. https://doi.org/10.1136/bmj.38142.554479.AE.

Durrant, G., & Goldstein, H. (2008). *Analysing The Probability Of Attrition In A Longitudinal Survey*. Retrieved from.

Gjonca, E., Tabassum, F., & Breeze, E. (2009). Socioeconomic differences in physical disability at older age. *Journal of Epidemiology and Community Health, 63*(11), 928–935. https://doi.org/10.1136/jech.2008.082776.

Greenland, S. (1996). Basic methods for sensitivity analysis of biases. *International Journal of Epidemiology, 25*(6), 1107–1116. https://doi.org/10.1093/ije/25.6.1107-a.

Groot, W. (2000). Adaptation and scale of reference bias in self-assessments of quality of life. *Journal of Health Economics, 19*(3), 403–420.

Grundy, E., & Sloggett, A. (2003). Health inequalities in the older population: The role of personal capital, social resources and socio-economic circumstances. *Social Science & Medicine, 56*(5), 935–947.

Harper, S., Lynch, J., Hsu, W.-L., Everson, S. A., Hillemeier, M. M., Raghunathan, T. E., ... Kaplan, G. A. (2002). Life course socioeconomic conditions and adult psychosocial functioning. *International Journal of Epidemiology, 31*(2), 395–403. https://doi.org/10.1093/ije/31.2.395.

Huisman, M., Kunst, A. E., & Mackenbach, J. P. (2003). Socioeconomic inequalities in morbidity among the elderly; a European overview. *Social Science & Medicine, 57*(5), 861–873.

Imai, K., Keele, L., & Tingley, D. (2010). A general approach to causal mediation analysis. *Psychological Methods, 15*(4), 309–334. https://doi.org/10.1037/a0020761.

Jivraj, S., Goodman, A., Ploubidis, G. B., & de Oliveira, C. (2017). Testing Comparability Between Retrospective Life History Data and Prospective Birth Cohort Study Data. *Journals of Gerontology Series B-Psychological Sciences and Social Sciences*. https://doi.org/10.1093/geronb/gbx042.

Kannel, W. B., & Sorlie, P. (1979). Some health benefits of physical-activity—Framingham-study. *Archives of Internal Medicine, 139*(8), 857–861. https://doi.org/10.1001/archinte.139.8.857.

Kaplan, G. A., Pamuk, E. R., Lynch, J. W., Cohen, R. D., & Balfour, J. L. (1996). Inequality in income and mortality in the United States: Analysis of mortality and potential pathways. *British Medical Journal, 312*(7037), 999–1003.

Kobayashi, L. C., Beeken, R. J., & Meisel, S. F. (2017). Biopsychosocial predictors of perceived life expectancy in a national sample of older men and women. *Plos One, 12*(12), e0189245. https://doi.org/10.1371/journal.pone.0189245.

Kuh, D. J., & Cooper, C. (1992). Physical activity at 36 years: Patterns and childhood predictors in a longitudinal study. *Journal of Epidemiology and Community Health, 46*(2), 114–119.

Leon, D. A., Saburova, L., Tomkins, S., McKee, M., & Shkolnikov, V. M. (2007). Alcohol consumption and public health in Russia. *Lancet, 370*(9587), 561–561. https://doi.org/10.1016/s0140-6736(07)61281-1.

Lindeboom, M., & van Doorslaer, E. (2004). Cut-point shift and index shift in self-reported health. *Journal of Health Economics, 23*(6), 1083–1099. https://doi.org/10.1016/j.jhealeco.2004.01.002. ISSN 0167-6296.

Little, R. J. A., & Rubin, D. B. (1989). The analysis of social-science data with missing values. *Sociological Methods & Research, 18*(2–3), 292–326.

Little, R. J. A., & Rubin, D. B. (2002). *Statistical analysis with missing data* (2nd ed.). Chichester: Willey.

Lynch, J. W., Kaplan, G. A., & Salonen, J. T. (1997). Why do poor people behave poorly? Variation in adult health behaviours and psychosocial characteristics by stages of the socioeconomic lifecourse. *Social Science & Medicine, 44*(6), 809–819. https://doi.org/10.1016/S0277-9536(96)00191-8.

Lynch, J. W., Smith, G. D., Kaplan, G. A., & House, J. S. (2000). Income inequality and mortality: Importance to health of individual income, psychosocial environment, or material conditions. *British Medical Journal, 320*(7243), 1200–1204.

Mackenbach, J., Stirbu, I., Roskam, A., Schaap, M., Menvielle, G., Leinsalu, M., & Kunst, A. (2008). Socioeconomic inequalities in health in 22 European countries. *New England Journal of Medicine, 358*, 2468–2481.

Mackenbach, J. P. (2012). The persistence of health inequalities in modern welfare states: The explanation of a paradox. *Social Science & Medicine, 75*(4), 761–769. https://doi.org/10.1016/j.socscimed.2012.02.031.

Marmot, M., Banks, J., Blundell, R., Lessof, C., & Nazroo, J. (Eds.). (2002). *Health, wealth and lifestyles of the older population in England: The 2002 English longitudinal study of ageing*. Institute for Fiscal Studies.

Ploubidis, G., DeStavola, B., & Grundy, E. (2011). Health differentials in the older population of England: An empirical comparison of the materialist, lifestyle and psychosocial hypotheses. *BMC Public Health, 11*(1), 390.

Ploubidis, G. B., Benova, L., Grundy, E., Laydon, D., & DeStavola, B. (2014). Lifelong Socio Economic Position and biomarkers of later life health: Testing the contribution of competing hypotheses. *Social Science & Medicine, 119*, 258–265. https://doi.org/10.1016/j.socscimed.2014.02.018.

Ploubidis, G. B., & Grundy, E. (2009). Later-life mental health in Europe: A country-level comparison. *Journals of Gerontology Series B-Psychological Sciences and Social Sciences, 64*(5), 666–676. https://doi.org/10.1093/geronb/gbp026.

Rabe-Hesketh, S., & Skrondal, A. (2008). Classical latent variable models for medical research. *Statistical Methods in Medical Research, 17*(1), 5–32. https://doi.org/10.1177/0962280207081236.

Rose, G. (1985). Sick individuals and sick populations. *International Journal of Epidemiology, 14*(1), 32–38. https://doi.org/10.1093/ije/14.1.32.

Schrijvers, C. T. M., Stronks, K., van de Mheen, H. D., & Mackenbach, J. P. (1999). Explaining educational differences in mortality: The role of behavioral and material factors. *American Journal of Public Health, 89*(4), 535–540.

Snowden, J. M., Rose, S., & Mortimer, K. M. (2011). Implementation of G-computation on a simulated data set: Demonstration of a causal inference technique. *American Journal of Epidemiology, 173*(7), 731–738. https://doi.org/10.1093/aje/kwq472.

Steptoe, A., Breeze, E., Banks, J., & Nazroo, J. (2012). Cohort profile: The English longitudinal study of ageing. *International Journal of Epidemiology*. https://doi.org/10.1093/ije/dys168.

Stringhini, S., Zaninotto, P., Kumari, M., Kivimäki, M., & Batty, G. D. (2016). Lifecourse socioeconomic status and type 2 diabetes: The role of chronic inflammation in the English longitudinal study of ageing. *Scientific Reports, 6*, 24780. https://doi.org/10.1038/srep24780, https://www.nature.com/articles/srep24780#supplementary-information.

Tammelin, T., Nayha, S., Hills, A. P., & Jarvelin, M. R. (2003). Adolescent participation in sports and adult physical activity. *American Journal of Preventive Medicine, 24*(1), 22–28.

Ten Have, T. R., & Joffe, M. M. (2012). A review of causal estimation of effects in mediation analyses. *Statistical Methods in Medical Research, 21*(1), 77–107. https://doi.org/10.1177/0962280210391076.

van de Mheen, H., Stronks, K., Looman, C., & Mackenbach, J. (1998). Does childhood socioeconomic status influence adult health through behavioural factors? *International Journal of Epidemiology, 27*(3), 431–437. https://doi.org/10.1093/ije/27.3.431.

Vanderweele, T. J. (2012). Mediation analysis with multiple versions of the mediatore. *Epidemiology (Cambridge, Massachusetts), 23*(3), 454–463.

Vanderweele, T. J., Vansteelandt, S., & Robins, J. M. (2014). Effect decomposition in the presence of an exposure-induced mediator-outcome confounder. *Epidemiology, 25*(2), 300–306. https://doi.org/10.1097/ede.0000000000000034.

Warburton, D. E. R., Nicol, C. W., & Bredin, S. S. D. (2006). Health benefits of physical activity: The evidence. *Canadian Medical Association Journal, 174*(6), 801–809. https://doi.org/10.1503/cmaj.051351.

Wardle, J., & Steptoe, A. (2003). Socioeconomic differences in attitudes and beliefs about healthy lifestyles. *Journal of Epidemiology and Community Health, 57*(6), 440–443. https://doi.org/10.1136/jech.57.6.440.

Chapter 3
Physical Activity: A Moderator or Mediator in the Association Between Fertility History and Later Life Health?

Sanna Read and Emily Grundy

Abstract Large family size and early parenthood have been associated with adverse health outcomes in old age whereas there is increasing evidence of the beneficial effects of physical activity. We examined the extent to which physical activity might mediate and/or moderate later life health disadvantages related to a high number of children and early parenthood. We used data from five waves of the English Longitudinal Study of Ageing collected in 2002–2010 ($n = 11{,}233$ in wave 1). Latent change score modelling was used to assess the direction of the association between physical activity and functioning. An interaction term of physical activity and fertility history was added in latent growth curves for functional limitation. The models were adjusted for age, gender, smoking, educational attainment, occupational status and wealth in wave 1, with whether married and depressive symptoms included as time-varying covariates. The models suggested that physical activity serves as a mediator in the association between fertility history and the level of later life functioning. However, there was no effect of fertility history on changes in physical activity or functional limitation. Among those who were physically active, functional limitations remained at a considerably lower level and high number of children and early parenthood were not associated with poorer levels of health. Physical activity thus moderates the level of health disadvantages related to high number of children and parenthood.

Keywords Physical activity · Fertility history · Later life health

---

S. Read (✉) · E. Grundy
London School of Economics and Political Science, London, UK
e-mail: s.read@lse.ac.uk

E. Grundy
e-mail: emily.grundy@essex.ac.uk

G. B. Ploubidis et al., *Pathways to Health*,
SpringerBriefs in Population Studies,
https://doi.org/10.1007/978-94-024-1707-4_3

3.1 Introduction

Physical activity has been associated with numerous advantageous health outcomes throughout the life course, including better survival (Woodcock, Franco, Orsini, & Roberts, 2011), and a lower risk of developing diseases (Vuillemin, 2012; Warburton, Nicol, & Bredin, 2006) and functional limitations (von Bonsdorff & Rantanen, 2011). Implementing physical exercise programmes has shown health improvements in many different groups of community dwelling older people and older patients (see for reviews Blake, Mo, Malik, & Thomas, 2009; Speck, Courneya, Masse, Duval, & Schmitz, 2010; Stuifbergen, Morris, Jung, Pierini, & Morgan, 2010).

While physical activity seems to be a powerful tool for improving health and well-being among various target populations, it is not clear whether it may interact with long-term health disadvantages related to life events earlier in the life cycle which, by definition, are fixed before the onset of older age. Some fertility history events, such as higher number of children and early childbirth are examples of life events experienced in the first half of life which have been shown to be related to later adverse outcomes Previous intervention studies focusing on the buffering effect of physical activity on fertility events have only studied the effects of exercise immediately after childbirth, ignoring the long-term effects in later life (Choi, Fukuoka, & Lee, 2013; Davenport, Giroux, Sopper, & Mottola, 2011; van der Pligt et al., 2013). While intervention studies in older age would be needed to fully answer the question of long-term effects, analyses of the moderating effects of physical activity in observational studies may provide useful information on the potential value of such studies and approaches.

Although evidence of the late life buffering effect of physical activity is scarce, there are previous studies showing associations between fertility history, physical activity and later life health. For instance, later life health disadvantages are associated with a higher number of children (high parity) and early timing of entry to parenthood (Grundy & Read, 2015; Grundy & Tomassini, 2005; Read, Grundy, & Wolf, 2011; Spence, 2008), although the results for high parity and functioning have been mixed in some studies (Aiken, Angel, & Miles, 2012; Henretta, 2007; Spence, 2008; Spence & Eberstein, 2009). Early parenthood may involve accumulated stresses related to lowered opportunities for education and career development and lower income and support networks (Spence, 2008). Compared to the childless, parents are more likely to adopt health promoting behaviours (Kendig, Dykstra, van Gaalen, & Melkas, 2007; Umberson, Crosnoe, & Reczek, 2010). However, among parents having a high number of children and early parenthood are associated with a less healthy life style (Umberson, Liu, Mirowsky, & Reczek, 2011). Over time these accumulated stresses (in this case lower educational level, disadvantageous fertility history and sedentary life style) may contribute to the development of physical dysfunction, disease and functional limitations (McEwen, 2003). In previous work we have shown that links between high parity and early parenthood and later life long-term illness that limited activities partly operated through education, physical activity, and physiological stress (Grundy & Read, 2015). However, this study did not assess the direction of the effect: it is possible that functional limitation may inhibit physical activity rather than other way round. It also did not measure dynamic associations with the rate of change in physical activity or functional limitations.

The previous evidence thus suggests that physical activity may act as a mediator and a moderator of the association between fertility history and later life functioning. In the present study we investigate whether physical activity mediates the association between a higher number of children and early parenthood and later life development of functional limitations and whether physical activity moderates the burden of functional limitations in later life related to high number of children and early parenthood. We use the English Longitudinal Study of Ageing (ELSA) which provides repeated measures over time making it possible not only to assess the direction and dynamic associations of these pathways (mediation) but also the possible main and interaction effect of the initial level to change (moderation).

3.2 Method

3.2.1 Sample

We use data from the English Longitudinal Study of Ageing, a nationally representative longitudinal study of the older population of England. The first wave of ELSA conducted in 2002–2003 included men and women then aged 50 years or more from private households which had participated in any one of the 1998, 1999 or 2001 rounds of the cross sectional Health Survey for England (HSE; an annual health survey based on a stratified random sample of all households in England). Response rates for the HSE were 69% in 1998, 70% in 1999 and 67% in 2001. This process led to the recruitment of 11,392 core members to the first wave of the ELSA study (response rate 67%). Of these, 11,233 provided in-person interviews and were included in this study. Comparisons with other sources, including the national census, showed that at baseline the ELSA survey was nationally representative. Respondents have been re-interviewed every two years. In the present study we use data from the five first waves to measure the level and rate of change in functional limitations over a 10-year-period. The number of respondents for each variable in the 5 waves are shown in Tables 3.1 and 3.2.

3.2.2 Measures

Functional limitations were measured using a count of self-reported difficulty in performing 10 tasks related to mobility, strength and endurance. These tasks were walking 100 yards, sitting for about two hours, getting up from a chair after sitting for long periods, climbing several flights of stairs without resting, climbing one flight

Table 3.1 Distributions of time-invariant variables at Wave 1

Variable	% or mean (SD)	*N*
Age in years (range 50–91[a])	65.2 (10.35)	11233
Male	45.5	11233
Educational qualification	57.4	11214
Occupational status		10770
Professional/managerial	31.9	
Skilled non-manual	24.1	
Skilled manual	20.4	
Unskilled or semi-skilled manual	23.6	
Net wealth quintile (range 1–5)	3.0 (1.41)	11134
Smoking status		11219
Never smoked	35.6	
Current smoker	17.8	
Past smoker	46.6	
Number of natural children		11233
0	15.6	
1	15.7	
2	38.3	
3	18.6	
4+	11.8	
Early parenthood[b]	12.9	

[a]Ages 91+ have been combined in one category to promote anonymity within the sample
[b]First birth at age <20 for mothers and <23 for fathers

of stairs without resting, stooping, kneeling and crouching, reaching or extending arms above shoulder level, pulling or pushing large objects like a living room chair, lifting or carrying weights over 10 lb, and picking up a 5 p coin from a table.

Self-reported *physical activity* was used to create three categories: Sedentary or mild (no physical activity or mild physical activity and, if working, in a sedentary job or in a job that was mostly standing); moderate (moderate physical activity at least once a week or, if working, in a job that involved physical work), and vigorous (vigorous physical activity at least once a week or, if working, in a job that involved heavy manual labour) (de Oliveira, Shankar, Kumari, Nunn, & Steptoe, 2010). The highest category was chosen as the indicator of being physically active and in the interaction model this category was compared against the other categories indicating lower physical activity. For the purpose of comparing the thresholds, the models were also fitted using two other cut-off points: (1) moderate intensity of physical

Table 3.2 Distribution of time-varying variables (% or mean and *SD*)

Variables	Wave 1	*n*	Wave 2	*n*	Wave 3	*n*	Wave 4	*n*	Wave 5	*n*
Functional limitations count		11219		8718		7488		6581		6201
0	42.3		40.2		40.1		39.3		38.6	
1	16.8		16.6		16.3		15.7		15.9	
2	9.9		10.8		11.1		11.7		11.0	
3	7.8		7.7		7.8		8.2		7.5	
4	5.7		6.3		5.8		6.1		6.0	
5	4.4		4.8		4.9		5.2		5.0	
6	3.7		4.1		4.1		4.2		4.6	
7	3.5		3.3		3.6		4.0		4.3	
8	3.0		3.1		3.0		2.9		3.4	
9	2.1		2.2		2.2		1.8		2.3	
10	0.8		0.7		1.1		0.9		1.3	
Physical activity	1.95	11218	1.98	8650	1.93	7490	1.90	6580	1.88	6202
Currently married	66.5	11231	64.6	8718	62.9	7491	61.1	6582	58.8	6203
Depressive symptoms, CES-D8 > 2	24.7	11040	25.0	8588	24.6	7304	24.5	6344	27.2	5890

[a]Only among parents

activity at least once a week or (2) moderate intensity of physical activity several times a week. Multiple group models were tested to find out at what level of physical activity fertility history was not associated with health disadvantages.

Number of children was measured by five binary variables indicating whether respondents had had 0, 1, 2, 3, or 4+ natural living children. For parents, dichotomous variables were derived indicating whether or not respondents had experienced *early parenthood,* defined as having had a biological child before the age of 20 for women or 23 for men. These cut points were chosen on the basis of the relevant previous literature and the distribution observed in the sample (Hobcraft, 2008; Read et al., 2011).

A number of previously identified covariates (see Grundy & Read, 2015) were used. *Age* was included as a continuous variable measured in years. *Education* was dichotomised distinguishing respondents with any formal qualification from those with no qualifications. *Occupational status* of respondents' current or last job was classified into professional or managerial; skilled non-manual; skilled manual; and unskilled or semiskilled manual groupings using the British occupational based social class scheme (Galobardes, Shaw, Lawlor, Lynch, & Smith, 2006). *Wealth* quintiles were calculated using non-pension wealth indicating financial, physical and housing wealth net of debts. *Smoking* status was measured using three dichotomous variables indicating whether the participant was currently smoking, was an ex-smoker or had never smoked. Age, education, occupational status, wealth and smoking were measured in wave 1 and treated as time invariant variables. *Being married* was a binary measure (currently married/have partner vs. not married/no partner). *Depressive symptoms* were assessed using an 8-item version of Centre for Epidemiologic Studies Depression Scale (CES-D). Because of a skewed distribution the CES-D score was dichotomized with a count of three or more symptoms being coded as indicative of depressive symptomology (Shankar, McMunn, Banks, & Steptoe, 2011).

3.2.3 Analysis

Analyses were carried out using the Mplus software version 7.11 (Muthén, 1998–2012). We used a latent change score model (McArdle & Hamagami, 2001) based on the structural equation framework for investigating the directions of the longitudinal associations between physical activity and functional limitation. The model includes a latent growth curve model part, which in the present study assessed initial level (intercept) and slope. The model also estimates a latent difference score between each measurement occasion, which can be used to assess the direction of associations, e.g. whether the poor level of physical activity predicts faster decline in functioning level or vice versa. For the moderating effect of physical activity we used latent growth curve modeling.

All models were first fitted separately for men and women, but because the associations were very similar, men and women were analysed together in the analysis (except for the analysis of different thresholds of physical activity where gender differences were found). The ELSA sample includes all older people living in the same household and this clustering, which was mostly due to inclusion of partners living together, was taken into account in the models. As already indicated, models were adjusted for age, education, occupation status, wealth, being married, depressive symptoms and smoking. Continuous covariates were centered to make the interpretation of the estimates easier. Because the measure of functional limitations was very skewed and based on the number of tasks for which the respondent reported difficulties, it was treated as a count in the analysis. In the mediation model, physical activity was used as a continuous variable. A dichotomous physical activity variable and number of children and early parenthood were used to create the interaction terms. The significance of interaction terms was tested using the Wald test. The Wald test follows the χ^2 test distribution with degrees of freedom defined as the number of parameters in the comparison. A significant p-value in Wald test indicates that the interaction term is needed in the model. To assess whether the different thresholds of physical activity made any difference, two multiple group models were tested. In the first multiple group analysis, the groups were sedentary or mild physical activity; moderate physical activity at least once a week; and vigorous activity at least once a week. In the second multiple group analysis, the groups were sedentary or mild activity; moderate activity several times a week; and vigorous activity at least once a week.

Maximum likelihood estimation with robust standard errors (MLR) was used to take into account any non-normality in the sample. Full information maximum likelihood was used. This method includes all respondents in the data regardless of whether they participated in the later waves or responded to all items. The approach uses the information on mean and variance of the missing proportion of the variables given other observed variables. Using full information maximum likelihood is less biased and more efficient than e.g. listwise or pairwise deletion or similar response pattern imputation (Enders & Bandalos, 2001).

3.3 Results

3.3.1 Descriptive Results

Table 3.1 shows the distributions of the time-invariant variables from Wave 1. Age was on average 65 years. Forty-six percent of the sample were men. Nearly 60% had an educational qualification. About a third had had a professional or managerial occupation, nearly a fourth had had a skilled manual or unskilled/semi-skilled manual occupation, and a fifth a skilled manual occupation. Under 20% were current smokers, and nearly half were past smokers. Most men and women had 2 children (which was the reference category). About 11% had a high number of children (4+ children). About 13% had experienced early parenthood.

Table 3.2 shows the distributions of time-varying variables. Forty-two percent did not report any functional limitations in wave 1. The functional limitations count increased over time. Most people engaged in moderate physical activity and there was a slight decrease in physical activity over the waves. Two-thirds of the sample was married in wave 1 but this proportion declined over the waves. About the fourth of the sample reported at least three depressive symptoms in wave 1, and this proportion slightly increased over the waves.

About a third of men and women reported vigorous physical activity in wave 1 (Table 3.3). Higher parity and early parenthood were associated with lower levels of physical activity.

Those with missing functional limitation data in the follow-up were more likely to be older, men, current smokers, less physically active and belong to a lower occupational level and wealth quintile in wave 1 (results not shown). They were also less likely to have qualifications and be married. They tended to have a lower number of children (less than 2 children) and a higher proportion had had an early entry to parenthood.

3.3.2 Latent Change Score Models for Assessing the Change Over Time in Physical Activity and Functional Limitation and the Direction of Association Between Them

Table 3.4 shows results for the univariate change score models for physical activity and functional limitations. The models indicate that there was considerable individual change over time (residual variance). However, only functional limitation showed decrease in the sample mean (intercept). Initial level of physical activity did not correlate with this change. For functional limitation, a higher initial level was associated with less change over time. All covariates were associated with the level of physical activity and functional limitation. The only exception was marital status, which did not have any effect when other socio-economic factors were included in the model. The associations showed that older age, being a women, lower educational level and wealth, current smoking, large family size (4+ children versus 2 children), early parenthood and depressive symptoms were associated with a lower level of physical activity and higher level of functional limitations. As expected manual occupation was associated with a higher level of functional limitation, but not with physical activity as the measure took into account physical activity at work.

In addition to level, some of the covariates were also associated with the growth parameter of physical activity and functional limitation: older age was associated with less change in physical activity. The lowest occupation status was to some extent associated with less change in physical activity. Being a current smoker predicted a faster increase in functional limitations.

Table 3.3 Parameter estimates (SE) for the univariate latent difference score models of physical activity and functional limitations in waves 1–5

	Physical activity			Functional limitations		
Variables	Est.	(SE)	*p*	Est.	(SE)	*p*
Intercepts						
Level	2.25	(0.034)	***	1.56	(0.061)	***
Growth	0.02	(0.196)		0.16	(0.025)	***
Residual variances						
Observed variable	0.32	(0.005)	***	1.43	(0.026)	***
Level	0.31	(0.009)	***	3.93	(0.084)	***
Growth	0.02	(0.002)	***	0.11	(0.007)	***
Correlation between level and growth	−0.02	(0.024)		−0.11	(0.045)	*
Effects of time-invariant covariates						
Age on level	−0.02	(0.001)	***	0.06	(0.002)	***
Age on growth	−0.005	(0.002)	*	−0.01	(0.001)	
No educational qualification on level	−0.14	(0.017)	***	0.28	(0.051)	***
No educational qualification on growth	0.00	(0.014)		0.00	(0.015)	
Occupational status on level (ref = Professional/managerial)						
Skilled non-manual	−0.10	(0.019)	***	0.03	(0.059)	
Skilled manual	−0.01	(0.021)		0.24	(0.005)	***
Unskilled or semi-skilled manual	−0.04	(0.022)		0.14	(0.067)	*
Occupational status on growth (ref = Professional/managerial)						
Skilled non-manual	0.01	(0.012)		−0.00	(0.016)	
Skilled manual	−0.02	(0.011)		0.00	(0.019)	
Unskilled or semi-skilled manual	−0.03	(0.012)	*	0.02	(0.020)	
Wealth on level	0.09	(0.006)	***	−0.28	(0.017)	***
Wealth on growth	0.00	(0.008)		−0.01	(0.005)	
Smoking on level (ref = never smoked)						
Current smoker	−0.12	(0.021)	***	0.29	(0.067)	***
Past smoker	−0.01	(0.016)		0.29	(0.045)	***
Smoking on growth (ref = never smoked)						
Current smoker	−0.03	(0.017)		0.09	(0.020)	***
Past smoker	0.00	(0.007)		−0.01	(0.013)	
N of natural children on level (ref = 2)						
0	−0.11	(0.022)	***	0.05	(0.062)	
1	−0.05	(0.021)	*	0.14	(0.064)	*

(continued)

Table 3.3 (continued)

	Physical activity			Functional limitations		
Variables	Est.	(SE)	*p*	Est.	(SE)	*p*
3	−0.02	(0.019)		0.07	(0.059)	
4+	−0.07	(0.025)	**	0.25	(0.077)	**
N of natural children on growth (ref = 2)						
0	0.01	(0.014)		0.03	(0.019)	
1	−0.01	(0.011)		−0.01	(0.018)	
3	−0.01	(0.009)		−0.02	(0.016)	
4+	−0.00	(0.013)		−0.00	(0.022)	
Early parenthood on level[a]	−0.10	(0.025)	***	0.32	(0.081)	***
Early parenthood on growth[a]	0.01	(0.016)		0.03	(0.022)	
Time-varying effects						
Being married/have partner Wave 1	0.01	(0.015)		0.06	(0.042)	
Wave 2	0.00	(0.016)		0.08	(0.040)	
Wave 3	0.00	(0.005)		0.02	0.0431	
Wave 4	0.00	(0.005)		−0.02	(0.046)	
Wave 5	0.00	(0.006)		0.05	(0.055)	
Depression Wave 1	−0.07	(0.004)	***	0.21	(0.011)	***
Wave 2	−0.06	(0.004)	***	0.20	(0.010)	***
Wave 3	−0.06	(0.004)	***	0.20	(0.011)	***
Wave 4	−0.07	(0.005)	***	0.17	(0.013)	***
Wave 5	−0.06	(0.004)	***	0.20	(0.015)	***

* $p < 0.05$, ** $p < 0.01$, *** $p < 0.001$
[a]First birth at age <20 for mothers and <23 for fathers

Because high parity and early parenthood were not associated with the growth parameter of functional limitation, the mediation model predicting the rate of change in functional limitations was not feasonable??. We therefore dropped the growth parameter and estimated cross-lagged associations between the level of physical activity and level of functional limitation. These estimates showed a bidirectional association: previous physical activity predicted later functional limitation level (estimate = −0.06, SE = 0.002, p > 0.001) and previous functional limitation predicted later physical activity level (estimate = −0.07, SE = 0.007, p > 0.001).

Table 3.4 The main effects (Model 1) and interactions (Model 2) between vigorous physical activity and parity on the level of functional limitations from latent growth curve models for all men and women

	Model 1	Model 2
Vigorous physical activity	−1.00***	−0.82***
Number of children		
0	−0.04	0.01
1	0.12	0.22**
3	0.10	0.18*
4	0.24***	0.39***
*Interaction vigorous physical activity*number of children*		
0	–	−0.15
1	–	−0.34**
3	–	−0.26**
4	–	−0.55***

* $p < 0.05$, ** $p < 0.01$, *** $p < 0.001$. Models adjusted for age, qualification, occupational status, wealth, smoking, currently married and depressive symptoms. Note. Linear slope of functional limitations was not associated with physical activity or number of children, models shown for initial level only

3.3.3 Latent Growth Curves for Testing the Effect of Interaction Between Fertility History and Physical Activity on Functional Limitation

We fitted a latent growth curve for functional limitations including two growth parameters: initial level (intercept) and linear slope. Quadratic slope turned out to be non-significant, so it was dropped from the final models (results not shown). We first fitted the models with main effects for all men and women (Model 1, Table 3.5). Being less than vigorously physically active and having four or more children compared to two children were associated with higher levels of functional limitations. In the next step (Model 2, Table 3.5), we added the interaction term vigorous physical activity * number of children to the model. The interaction was significant, and removing the interaction terms would have reduced the fit of the model significantly (Wald test 20.31 ($df = 4$), $p < 0.001$). There was no evidence of interaction on the linear slope of functional limitation.

For parents, we fitted a model including the early parenthood variable. Early parenthood predicted a higher level of functional limitations (Model 1, Table 3.5). The interaction between vigorous physical activity and early child parenthood was significant (Model 2, Table 3.6). Removing it would have reduced the fit of the model significantly (Wald test 13.19 ($df = 1$), $p < 0.001$). There was no evidence of an interaction on the linear slope of functional limitation.

Table 3.5 The main effects (Model 1) and interaction (Model 2) between vigorous physical activity and early parenthood on the level of functional limitations in latent growth curve models for parous men and women

	Model 1	Model 2
Vigorous physical activity	−1.00***	−0.93***
Early parenthood	0.34***	0.50***
Interaction Vigorous physical activity*Early parenthood	–	−0.55***

* $p < 0.05$, ** $p < 0.01$, *** $p < 0.001$, [a]first birth at age <20 for mothers and <23 for fathers. Models adjusted for age, qualification, occupational status, wealth, smoking, currently married, number of children and depressive symptoms. Note. Linear slope of functional limitations was not associated with physical activity or number of children, models shown for initial level only

We illustrate the modification effect of vigorous physical activity on the association between number of children and level of functional limitations in Fig. 3.1. Those reporting vigorous physical activity had considerably lower levels of functional limitations throughout the follow-up. Among the vigorously physically active, number of children was not associated with any difference in functional limitations, whereas there was a clear disadvantage of high parity among the less physically active. In both the vigorously physically active and less active groups functional limitations

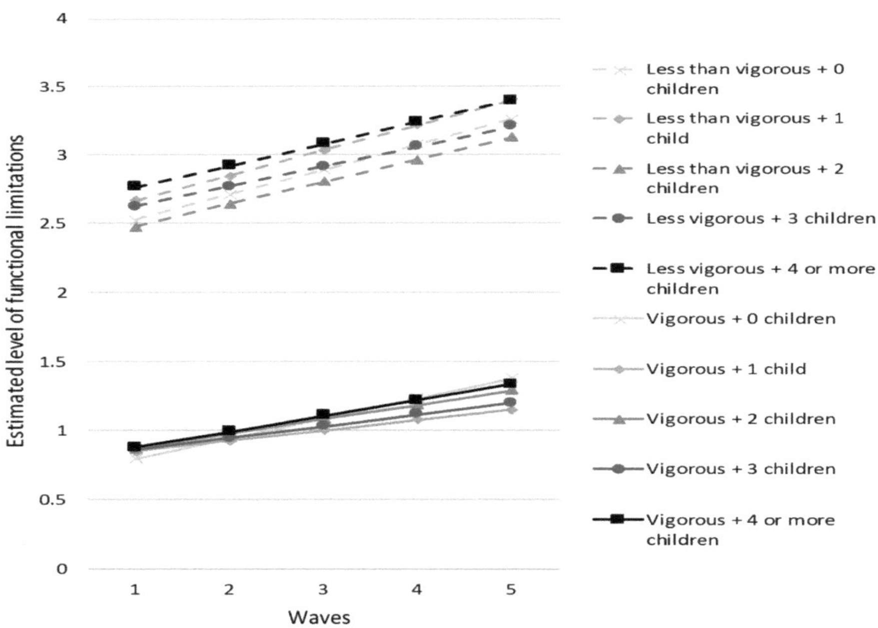

Fig. 3.1 The association between number of children and initial level of functional limitations modified by vigorous physical activity

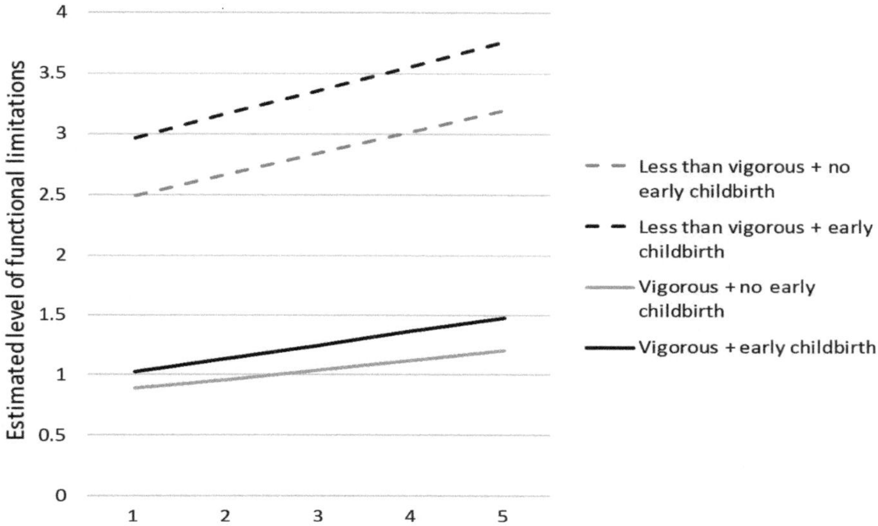

Fig. 3.2 The association between early parenthood and initial level of functional limitations modified by vigorous physical activity

increased over time. Experiencing early parenthood had very little effect on functional limitations among those who were vigorously physically active, whereas among the physically less active, early parenthood was associated with a considerably higher level of functional limitations (Fig. 3.2).

To assess whether lower intensity of physical activity could also moderate the association between fertility history and functional limitations, we tested models including a group for those who were not vigorously active, but were moderately physically active at least once a week or alternatively moderately active several times a week. The model also included the groups for those who reported vigorous physical activity at least once a week and those who reported being sedentary or taking mild, but not any moderate or vigorous, activity. The results indicated that in women moderate physical activity several times a week had a similar moderating effect as vigorous physical activity once a week (results not shown). Moderate activity once a week, however, did not moderate the association between fertility history and functional limitations. In men, moderate activity once or several times a week did not moderate the association between fertility history and functional limitations.

3.4 Discussion

We found evidence of both mediation and moderation between fertility history, physical activity and later life functional limitation. Early parenthood and a large family size were associated with lower physical activity in later life, which in turn predicted a higher level of functional limitations. Although the results supported the pathway presented in the previous path analysis (Grundy & Read, 2015), they also point to the fact that the association between level of physical activity and functional limitation is bidirectional. Therefore, the models are improved if they take into account repeated measures of both physical activity and functional limitation. Moreover, even though lower physical activity predicted a faster increase in functional limitation, the rate of change was not associated with high parity or early parenthood. This suggests that the association may be established in earlier life.

The interaction between fertility history and later life physical activity on functional limitation showed that vigorous physical activity at least once a week, and in women also moderate activity several times a week, may alleviate adverse health outcomes related to high parity and early parenthood. Current physical activity has been shown to be a powerful intervention tool to tackle health disadvantages (Blake et al., 2009; Speck et al., 2010; Stuifbergen et al., 2010). Physical activity can contribute to short-term health improvements around the time of transition to parenthood (Choi et al., 2013; Davenport et al., 2011; van der Pligt et al., 2013). The current results suggest that physical activity could also be useful later in life, although the effect only on the level suggests that there may be some relatively stable patterns related to health behaviours and their association with functioning. The current study cannot separate the effect of possible selection for instance into certain fertility, physical activity or health trajectories. More research is needed on the effects of life-time physical activity on later life activity levels and effects on functional limitation.

The results suggest that a relatively low frequency of vigorous activity, in this case vigorous activity at least once a week, is enough to modify the effect of high number of children and early parenthood on adverse health outcomes. Moreover, moderate activity several times a week moderated the association between fertility history and functional limitations in women, suggesting somewhere in between the moderate activity several times a week and moderate activity once a week there lies a threshold that makes the difference. In men, the threshold seemed to be higher (between vigorous activity once a week and moderate activity several times a week). In future studies it would be preferable to use a more finely graded scale (e.g. MET scores) to identify the threshold level of activity that starts to make a difference. Recent findings highlight the importance of focusing on lower frequencies and intensities as they in some cases result in significant improvements in health (Powell, Paluch, & Blair, 2011). In terms of functional limitations reduction, moderate amounts of activity are usually needed to improve functioning in older age (Physical, Activity, Guidelines, Advisory, & Committee, 2008).

Our results come from an observational study and there are some limitations in the measures and methods available to us. Physical activity was self-reported and it may be that differential over- or under-estimation of activity might bias results. As discussed above, physical activity in later life is likely to be correlated with physical activity earlier in life. It is possible that it is the later activity (or the most current), rather than the former, that is important. Although a number of socio-demographic factors and depressive symptoms were controlled for, there may still be a number of factors, such as motivation and personality characteristics, that are important for adherence to physical activity and health outcomes and are associated with fertility histories. It is not clear why some people are more prone to be physically active. In fact, a number of exercise referral schemes have shown great individual variability leading to no improvement at group-level (Pavey et al., 2011). This may be even more likely in the case of understanding the role of physical activity in long-term health trajectories.

It is noteworthy that early parenthood and high parity are themselves associated with lower levels of physical activity. On one hand this may make these subgroups an attractive target for interventions, as the advantage of increasing activity levels may prove to be proportionally more beneficial in sedentary subpopulations (Rhodes, Mark, & Temmel, 2012). On the other hand, these groups may have a long history of an inactive life style that may be very hard to break. This calls for more understanding of individual characteristics, such as personality and motivation, and the role of other environmental risk factors. At the moment the literature on the determinants of physical activity is inconclusive (Baert, Gorus, Mets, Geerts, & Bautmans, 2011; Koeneman, Verheijden, Chinapaw, & Hopman-Rock, 2011), and the role of the individual and environmental factors over the life course needs further study.

In summary, in the English population, early parenthood and large family size are associated with more sedentary behavior, lower physical activity is in turn associated with a higher level of functional limitations. Physical activity may have the potential to alleviate the long-term health disadvantages related to early parenthood and high number of children, but factors underlying the individual choices of active lifestyle and life time history of health-related behaviors are important to understand in developing interventions for these subgroups.

References

Aiken, A. R. A., Angel, J. L., & Miles, T. P. (2012). Pregnancy as a risk factor for ambulatory limitation in later life. *American Journal of Public Health, 102,* 2330–2335.

Baert, V., Gorus, E., Mets, T., Geerts, C., & Bautmans, I. (2011). Motivators and barriers for physical activity in the oldest old: A systematic review. *Ageing Research Reviews, 10,* 464–474.

Blake, H., Mo, P., Malik, S., & Thomas, S. (2009). How effective are physical activity interventions for alleviating depressive symptoms in older people? A systematic review. *Clinical Rehabilitation, 23,* 873–887.

Choi, J., Fukuoka, Y., & Lee, J. H. (2013). The effects of physical activity and physical activity plus diet interventions on body weight in overweight or obese women who are pregnant or in postpartum: A systematic review and meta-analysis of randomized controlled trials. *Preventive Medicine, 56,* 351–364.

Davenport, M. H., Giroux, I., Sopper, M. M., & Mottola, M. F. (2011). Postpartum exercise regardless of intensity improves chronic disease risk factors. *Medicine and Science in Sports and Exercise, 43,* 951–958.

de Oliveira, C., Shankar, A., Kumari, M., Nunn, S., & Steptoe, A. (2010). Health risk and health protective biological measures in later life. In J. Banks, C. Lessof, J. Nazroo, N. Rogers, M. Stafford, & A. Steptoe (Eds.), *Financial circumstances, health and well-being of the older popu-*

lation in England: The 2008 English Longitudinal Study of Ageing (pp. 275–347). London: The Institute of Fiscal Studies.
Enders, C. K., & Bandalos, D. L. (2001). The relative performance of full information maximum likelihood estimation for missing data in structural equation models. *Structural Equation Modeling-a Multidisciplinary Journal, 8,* 430–457.
Galobardes, B., Shaw, M., Lawlor, D. A., Lynch, J. W., & Smith, G. D. (2006). Indicators of social position (part 2). *Journal of Epidemiology and Community Health, 60,* 95–101.
Grundy, E., & Read, S. (2015). Pathways from fertility history to later life health: Results from analyses of the English Longitudinal Study of Ageing. *Demographic Research, 32*(4), 107–146.
Grundy, E., & Tomassini, C. (2005). Fertility history and health in later life: A record linkage study in England and Wales. *Social Science and Medicine, 61,* 217–228.
Henretta, J. C. (2007). Early childbearing, marital status, and women's health and mortality after age 50. *Journal of Health and Social Behavior, 48,* 254–266.
Hobcraft, J. (2008). The timing and partnership context of becoming a parent: Cohort and gender commonalities and differences in childhood antecedents. *Demographic Research, 19,* 1281–1322.
Kendig, H., Dykstra, P. A., van Gaalen, R. I., & Melkas, T. (2007). Health of aging parents and childless individuals. *Journal of Family Issues, 28,* 1457–1486.
Koeneman, M. A., Verheijden, M. W., Chinapaw, M. J. M., & Hopman-Rock, M. (2011). Determinants of physical activity and exercise in healthy older adults: A systematic review. *International Journal of Behavioral Nutrition and Physical Activity, 8,* 142.
McArdle, J. J., & Hamagami, F. (2001). Linear dynamic analyses of incomplete longitudinal data. In L. Collins & A. Sayer (Eds.), *Methods for the analysis of change* (pp. 137–176). Washington, DC: American Psychological Association.
McEwen, B. S. (2003). Interacting mediators of allostasis and allostatic load: Towards an understanding of resilience in aging. *Metabolism-Clinical and Experimental, 52,* 10–16.
Muthén, L. K., & Muthén. B. O. (1998–2012). *Mplus user's guide*. Los Angeles, CA: Muthén & Muthén.
Pavey, T. G., Anokye, N., Taylor, A. H., Trueman, P., Moxham, T., Fox, K. R., et al. (2011). The clinical effectiveness and cost-effectiveness of exercise referral schemes: A systematic review and economic evaluation. *Health Technology Assessment, 15,* 1–254.
Physical, Activity, Guidelines, Advisory, & Committee. (2008). *Physical activity guidelines advisory committee report. Part G, Section 6: Functional health.* Washington, DC: US Department of Health and Human Services. http://www.health.gov/paguidelines/Report/pdf/CommitteeReport.pdf.
Powell, K. E., Paluch, A. E., & Blair, S. N. (2011). Physical activity for health: What kind? How much? How intense? on top of what? In J. E. Fielding, R. C. Brownson & L. W. Green (Eds.), *Annual Review of Public Health, 32,* 349–365.
Read, S., Grundy, E., & Wolf, D. A. (2011). Fertility history, health, and health changes in later life: A panel study of British women and men born 1923–49. *Population Studies-a Journal of Demography, 65,* 201–215.
Rhodes, R. E., Mark, R. S., & Temmel, C. P. (2012). Adult sedentary behavior a systematic review. *American Journal of Preventive Medicine, 42*(3), E3–E28. https://doi.org/10.1016/j.amepre.2011.10.020.
Shankar, A., McMunn, A., Banks, J., & Steptoe, A. (2011). Loneliness, social isolation, and behavioral and biological health indicators in older adults. *Health Psychology, 30,* 377–385.
Speck, R. M., Courneya, K. S., Masse, L. C., Duval, S., & Schmitz, K. H. (2010). An update of controlled physical activity trials in cancer survivors: A systematic review and meta-analysis. *Journal of Cancer Survivorship-Research and Practice, 4,* 87–100.
Spence, N. J. (2008). The long-term consequences of childbearing physical and psychological well-being of mothers in later life. *Research on Aging, 30,* 722–751.
Spence, N. J., & Eberstein, I. W. (2009). Age at first birth, parity, and post-reproductive mortality among white and black women in the US, 1982–2002. *Social Science and Medicine, 68,* 1625–1632.

Stuifbergen, A. K., Morris, M., Jung, J. H., Pierini, D., & Morgan, S. (2010). Benefits of wellness interventions for persons with chronic and disabling conditions: A review of the evidence. *Disability and Health Journal, 3,* 133–145.

Umberson, D., Crosnoe, R., & Reczek, C. (2010). Social relationships and health behavior across the life course. *Annual Review of Sociology, 36,* 139–157.

Umberson, D., Liu, H., Mirowsky, J., & Reczek, C. (2011). Parenthood and trajectories of change in body weight over the life course. *Social Science and Medicine, 73,* 1323–1331.

van der Pligt, P., Willcox, J., Hesketh, K. D., Ball, K., Wilkinson, S., Crawford, D., et al. (2013). Systematic review of lifestyle interventions to limit postpartum weight retention: Implications for future opportunities to prevent maternal overweight and obesity following childbirth. *Obesity Reviews, 14,* 792–805.

von Bonsdorff, M. B., & Rantanen, T. (2011). Progression of functional limitations in relation to physical activity: A life course approach. *European Review of Aging and Physical Activity, 8,* 23–30.

Vuillemin, A. (2012). Benefits of physical activity on health among elderly. *Science & Sports, 27,* 249–253.

Warburton, D. E. R., Nicol, C. W., & Bredin, S. S. D. (2006). Health benefits of physical activity: The evidence. *Canadian Medical Association Journal, 174,* 801–809.

Woodcock, J., Franco, O. H., Orsini, N., & Roberts, I. (2011). Non-vigorous physical activity and all-cause mortality: Systematic review and meta-analysis of cohort studies. *International Journal of Epidemiology, 40,* 121–138.

Chapter 4
Self-rated Health Over the Life Course: Evidence from the 1958 and 1970 British Birth Cohorts

George B. Ploubidis and Benedetta Pongiglione

Abstract The twentieth century rise in life expectancy is undoubtedly one of the great successes of public health, but in combination with low fertility rates has also contributed importantly to the aging of populations. Population ageing poses great challenges and there is an urgent need for strategies to be developed that will help to alleviate its societal consequences. The proposed work focuses on one promising approach: achieving a 'compression of morbidity', or a reduction of the number of years spent in ill health. For a given level of life expectancy, a 'compression of morbidity' into a smaller number of years at the end of life would enable people to stay at work for a longer period of time, and also to care for themselves at advanced ages. In this chapter we investigated the progress of self-rated health over the life course in two well characterised population based representative British birth cohorts. The evolution of self-rated health over time differed between the two cohorts, both with respect to the shape of change over time as well as the average level of reported self-rated health. In the earlier born 1958 cohort self-rated health exhibited an almost linear trend with increasingly worse self-rated health being reported by both men and women as they moved from early adulthood to early old age. A different pattern was observed in the later born 1970 cohort, where the average level of self-ratted health remained stable up to age 34, but steadily declined from age 38 onwards in both men and women. In both men and women, the two cohorts reported similar level of self-rated health in early adulthood, but the trend diverged at age 42, where the 1970 cohort reported their health being significantly worse. Our observation of similar up to age 34 and then worse average self-rated health in the 1970 cohort increases the likelihood of expansion of morbidity, assuming that the observed difference as well as the lower mortality rates in the 1970 cohort will persist in the future.

G. B. Ploubidis (✉)
Centre for Longitudinal Studies, UCL Institute of Education, University College London, London, UK
e-mail: G.Ploubidis@UCL.ac.uk

B. Pongiglione
Milano, Italy
e-mail: benedetta.pongiglione@unibocconi.it

G. B. Ploubidis et al., *Pathways to Health*,
SpringerBriefs in Population Studies,
https://doi.org/10.1007/978-94-024-1707-4_4

Keywords Compression of morbidity · Population health change · Self-rated health

4.1 Introduction

The 20th century witnessed significant improvements in health in most countries including substantial increases in survival to older ages and large reductions in late age mortality (Leon, 2011). Life expectancy at birth in the United Kingdom (UK) increased by more than 30 years for both men and women, whereas in other high income countries it almost doubled ("Human Mortality Database," 2015; Leon, 2011; Mackenbach & Looman, 2013). This rapid and unprecedented increase in human life expectancy was associated with profound changes in the prevailing patterns of disease and morbidity, the so-called 'epidemiological transition'(Omran, 1971). Chronic illnesses, especially cancers and diseases of the circulatory system, replaced infectious diseases as the leading causes of death, while the risk of dying at earlier ages fell dramatically resulting in a postponement of death to older ages. The twentieth century rise in life expectancy is undoubtedly one of the great successes of public health, but in combination with low fertility rates has also contributed importantly to the aging of western populations. Ageing poses great challenges to the modern welfare state, not only by threatening the sustainability of pension systems but also by inducing a greater demand for social services, including healthcare. Although several factors underlie the increase in healthcare costs, aging is an important driver of this increase in the long run (Polder, Barendregt, & van Oers, 2006; Werblow, Felder, & Zweifel, 2007; Zweifel, Felder, & Meiers, 1999). There is therefore an urgent need for developing strategies that help to alleviate the societal consequences of population ageing. If the association between age and ill health is seen as immutable, then population ageing will inevitably lead to higher rates of morbidity, disability, and demand for healthcare and other social services. However this need not be the case, as evidence suggests that many manifestations of ill health at advanced ages are amenable to intervention, such as prevention by lifestyle modification, detection at earlier stages of life, treatment or rehabilitation (Khaw, 1997; Peres, Jagger, Matthews, & Mrc, 2008). Not only mortality can be postponed, as reflected in the increase of life expectancy, but the onset of morbidity can also be postponed (Fries, 2005).

This rapid increase in life expectancy has raised the question of how healthily the gained years of life will be spent. A pertinent question concerns the effect of the continuing postponement of death from chronic degenerative disease on the experience of the successive birth cohorts that will eventually make up the older population. How do the more recent cohorts compare with the earlier cohorts? Are the additional years of life that the most recent cohorts have gained (and stand to gain) years of good health or years of disability and frailty? In other words, are younger (more recently born) cohorts healthier compared to older (earlier born) cohorts? There are three theories focusing on the past and possible future developments of mortality and morbidity that attempt to predict how the added years will be lived. Each theory has different assumptions and different implications for the period of morbidity and disability at the end of life. The three theories are: (i) Compression of Morbidity; (ii) Expansion of Morbidity; (iii) Dynamic equilibrium. Each theory highlights one causal driver for the observed decline in mortality rates in old age and provides us with a view of what to expect with respect to the number of years lived in good health as mortality rates continue to fall and—consequently—life expectancy is rising. Gaining more understanding of the mechanisms that increase the likelihood of each scenario, in other words whether longer survival is accompanied by expansion, compression or dynamic equilibrium of morbidity is urgently needed. This has implications for the development of health systems in terms of costs, design and focus of public health and prevention policies.

The three theories are depicted in Graph 4.1, where a typical scenario of a hypothetical high income/low mortality country is presented: In row (A) the life expectancy of the country (80 years) on time "t" is depicted. Morbidity has an average onset at age 50 and the average time spent with morbidity is 30 years. The years lived in good health are depicted with the Cambridge blue bar, whereas the red bar denotes the number of years after the onset of morbidity. The Compression of Morbidity hypothesis is presented in row (B), where life expectancy in time (t + 30 years) has risen to 90 years and the average onset of morbidity to age 70. We see that the average time spent with morbidity has now decreased ("compressed") to 20 years and the years lived in good health have increased to 70 years. In its original form the compression of morbidity theory was proposed by Fries (1980), Fries, Bruce, & Chakravarty (2011) who argued that the onset of chronic diseases will be postponed, assuming that the average maximum life span will not exceed 85 years and morbidity would then be compressed into a shorter period of time at the end of life. If we suppose that increases in life expectancy are driven mainly by changes in underlying patterns of disease (people are living longer because the onset of chronic degenerative disease is being delayed to later ages), then we should expect to see a compression of morbidity provided that the observed increases in life expectancy are slowing down. General health improvements lead to increasing life expectancy and the impact of such health improvements on total life expectancy is hypothesised to diminish as human longevity approaches its natural limits.

However, it is well known by now that life expectancy has exceeded 85 years in Japan (Yong & Saito, 2009) and that in other high income countries its increase shows no signs of slowing down ("Human Mortality Database," 2015; David A. Leon, 2011; Oeppen & Vaupel, 2002). Fortunately, even if life expectancy continues to rise at the same rate, compression can be achieved if healthy life expectancy grows even faster. A necessary condition for this scenario to occur is that the onset of morbidity is postponed/delayed in younger/more recently born cohorts. In other words for compression to occur, younger cohorts that are expected to live longer have to be healthier compared to older/earlier born cohorts. It follows that younger cohorts being healthier becomes a sufficient condition for compression of morbidity if the observed increase in life expectancy slows down (stagnates) or stops. Compressing morbidity into a smaller number of years at the end of life would enable people to stay at work for a longer period of time, to care for themselves at advanced ages,

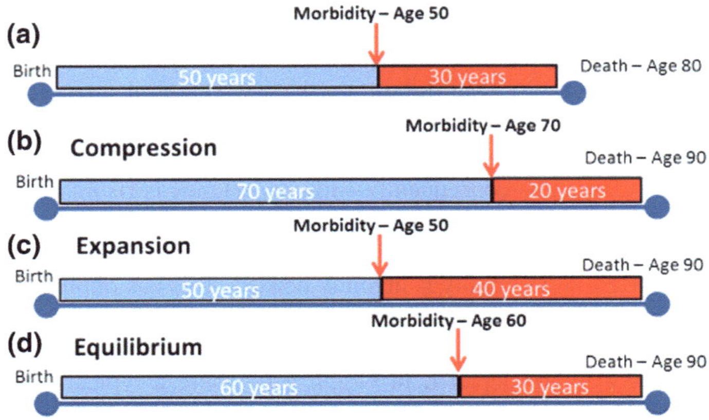

Graph 4.1 Compression, expansion and dynamic equilibrium hypotheses for a hypothetical population

enhance their well-being and reduce the demand for health services. Healthy ageing (Khaw, 1997) therefore depends on whether compression will be achieved and more research to inform interventions that can make this possible is urgently needed.

The Expansion of Morbidity theory (Gruenberg, 1977; Olshansky, Rudberg, Carnes, Cassel, & Brody, 1991) is depicted in row (C) of Graph 4.1. Life expectancy at (t + 30) has risen to 90 years, but the average age of onset of morbidity remained stable at 50 years. This has resulted in an expansion (increase) of the average years spent with morbidity to 40 years. In this scenario, total life expectancy is growing at a faster rate compared to healthy life expectancy, younger/more recently born cohorts have similar health (same average onset of morbidity) compared to older/earlier born cohorts and consequently the years lived with morbidity expand. According to this theory, expansion is mostly due to medical advances that push down the mortality rates of the major drivers of mortality such as cardiovascular disease, stroke and cancer after diagnosis while their average age of onset stays more or less the same. According to this scenario of the joint progress of health and mortality people will survive for longer with chronic illness, and as a consequence, the period of time that people spend in a state of chronic ill-health and disability at the end of life will increase. The original expansion of morbidity theory highlighted the implications for population health of the increasing capabilities of science and modern medicine to prevent death in people with fairly severe and potentially fatal chronic disease (Gruenberg, 1977; Olshansky et al., 1991). It also assumed that the underlying pathology and epidemiology of these chronic degenerative diseases is so closely related to the ageing process that it would remain resistant to the best efforts of medical technology and improvements in public health.

The third hypothesis—Dynamic Equilibrium-proposed by Manton (1982) suggests a continuation of the status quo, where the increase in life expectancy which assumes a continuing decline of mortality rates is accompanied by an equivalent postponement of the onset of morbidity. The theory is presented in Row D: Life expectancy has increased 10 years and has reached age 90, but the onset of morbidity has also been postponed by 10 years to age 60. This has resulted in 30 years lived with morbidity, as in time (t) where life expectancy was 80 years. An alternative interpretation suggests that dynamic equilibrium occurs when the years spent with mild or moderate disability expand, but years spent with severe disability compress (Jagger et al., 2017). This theory might at first glance appear appealing as it would have less negative consequences compared to an expansion of morbidity. However, if realised, this scenario will still increase the burden on the health care system despite the stabilisation of the years lived with morbidity, since due to population ageing more people will be surviving in 30 year period at (t + 30) compared to (t).

Whether longer survival is accompanied by expansion, compression or equilibrium of morbidity has therefore profound implications for the development of health systems in terms of costs and design as well as for the focus of public health policy. There is clearly scope for healthy ageing only if compression of morbidity is achieved, since improvements in population health and consequent increases in healthy life expectancy are not enough if they are not accompanied by compression. To achieve absolute compression in a population, younger/more recently born cohorts have to be healthier than older/earlier born cohorts, so the average onset of morbidity is postponed and healthy life expectancy increases faster than total life expectancy. Although this goal is ambitious, enormous potential exists for making substantial progress. If compression is achieved, it would reduce the cost of health services, enable people to stay at work for a longer period of time, and also to care for themselves at advanced ages. It is therefore of great importance to know whether the period of morbidity and disability at the end of life is increasing (expansion of morbidity), decreasing (compression) or staying more or less the same (equilibrium). Crucially, we also want to know which policy modifiable factors lead to compression of morbidity, the only scenario that has the potential to offset the effects of population ageing.

Surprisingly, despite its obvious importance for public health policy, the relative progression of morbidity and mortality is a relatively under-researched area, with the evidence for the three theories being mixed. Results from the latest Global Burden of Disease Study and recent evidence from the US point to an expansion of morbidity (Crimmins & Beltran-Sanchez, 2011; Crimmins, Zhang, & Saito, 2016; Salomon et al., 2012), in contrast to evidence from Europe (Cambois, Robine, & Hayward, 2001; Hessler et al., 2003) and the US where a compression of morbidity is suggested (Manton, 2008; Manton, Stallard, & Corder, 1998) (Crimmins, Saito, & Kim, 2016). The mixed evidence is at least partly due to the fact that in most studies single indicators of health or disability have been used and the question of whether expansion, compression or equilibrium is supported depends partly on the health indicator employed. For example, when using self-reported disability, the increase in life expectancy is more likely to lead to an expansion of morbidity (Crimmins, Saito, & Ingegneri, 1997; Robine & Mathers, 1993), whereas studies that analyse self-rated health usually tend to find a compression of morbidity (van de Water, Boshuizen, & Perenboom, 1996; Waidmann, Bound, & Schoenbaum, 1995).

In the UK the prevalence of severe functional limitations reported in 1994 were higher compared to 1988 (Grundy & Glaser, 2000), while between 1980 and 1994 there seemed to be an increase in disability-free life expectancy for females age 65 (Bebbington & Darton, 1996) and handicap-free life expectancy increased between 1976 and 1991, but the trend reversed downwardly between 1991 and 1994 (J.-M. Robine, Romieu, & Cambois, 1999). The most recent evidence (Jagger et al., 2016) shows that during the past two decades in England, cognitive impairment compressed in absolute terms (i.e. supporting evidence of reduction), self-perceived health compressed in relative terms (i.e. increase in the proportion of life spent healthy), and disability evolved in dynamic equilibrium, and disentangling its trends, less severe disability was found to increase but more severe disability was not.

A major limitation of the existing literature is that with a few exceptions in Europe and the US (Fries, 1996; Hubert, Bloch, Oehlert, & Fries, 2002; Nusselder, Looman, van de Mheen, van de Mheen, & Mackenbach, 2000), there is a complete lack of evidence on the factors that lead to compression, expansion or dynamic equilibrium. The life course perspective offers a unique opportunity to explore the causal processes that underlie the relative progress of morbidity and mortality and lead to compression, expansion or dynamic equilibrium in later life. This approach encompasses ideas and observations from an array of disciplines, notably history, sociology, demography, developmental psychology, biology, and economics. In particular, it directs attention to the powerful connection between individual lives and the historical and socioeconomic context in which these lives unfold (Giele & Elder, 1998). In this chapter we employ between cohort comparisons as an empirical tool to test the likelihood of the compression, expansion and dynamic equilibrium hypotheses. Between cohort comparisons with respect to health status at fixed ages over the life course is an innovative research design within which the three hypotheses can be empirically tested. Taking into account that due to increases in life expectancy younger (more recently born) cohorts are expected to live longer, a necessary condition for compression of morbidity is that after controlling for age differences, younger cohorts are healthier compared to older cohorts, so the average onset of morbidity is postponed. On the contrary, given the observed decline in mortality rates, expansion will invariably occur if younger cohorts are less healthy compared to older/earlier born cohorts, whereas similar health levels between cohorts will most likely lead to dynamic equilibrium. Considering the abundance of evidence which suggests that health at earlier stages in the life course has a strong effect on later life health (Birnie et al., 2011; Birnie et al., 2011; Cooper, Strand, Hardy, Patel, & Kuh, 2014; Kuh & Ben-Shlomo, 2004; Kuh, Ben-Shlomo, Lynch, Hallqvist, & Power, 2003; Leon et al., 1998), therefore influencing the cohort specific average onset of morbidity, it is safe to assume that between cohort health differences observed in mid-life will propagate or even expand in later life unless some intervention that aims to reverse these takes place. We employed two well characterised prospective population based British birth cohorts in order to compare the health status of individuals born in 1958 and 1970 at ages 23–55. Capitalising on the availability of comparable self-reported health indicators for the two cohorts at fixed ages in mid-life we empirically test whether the joint progress of health and mortality in these two generations support the expansion, compression or dynamic equilibrium hypotheses.

4.2 Methods

4.2.1 Data

We employed two nationally representative British birth cohorts: (i) The National Child Development Study (NCDS) (Power & Elliott, 2006) is the second oldest of the British cohort studies, with 10 major follow-ups since birth. The initial sample of 17,415 individuals—consisting of all babies born in Great Britain in a single week in 1958—are now approaching 60 years of age (most recent follow-up at age 55, age 61 sweep to commence in 2019), providing high quality prospective data on social, biological, physical, and psychological phenotypes at every sweep. (ii) The 1970 British Cohort Study (BCS70) (Waynforth, 2012) (www.cls.ioe.ac.uk) is a cohort study of all babies born in Great Britain in a single week in 1970. The initial sample of 16,569 individuals have been surveyed at 8 major sweeps, most recently in 2012 (age 42) when 9,066 of the study members were interviewed in person. The latest major phase of data collection took place in 2016 and continued to 2017 (age 46–47). This will be the study's first full adult biomedical sweep, including physical measurements, cognitive assessments and collection of blood samples.

4.2.2 Measures

Self-reported measures of health typically include self-rated general health status, reported presence of longstanding illness, self-reported problems with functional activities and, in some studies, self-report of particular conditions or symptoms (Bowling, 1995), with self-rated health being the most widely used health indicator in population surveys (DeSalvo, Bloser, Reynolds, He, & Muntner, 2006). Self-assessment of health is an easy to use measure and has been shown to strongly predict mortality (DeSalvo et al., 2006; Idler & Benyamini, 1997) even when other measures of current health, such as chronic illness, functional limitations, as well as objective are statistically controlled. These results have been replicated in several cultures (Jylha, Guralnik, Ferruci et al. 1998), age-groups (Grant, Piotrowski & Chappell 1995), and have led researchers worldwide to consider self-rated health an important research tool in monitoring population health.

In this study we employ the "traditional" self-rated health item which has been included in both surveys in similar format. In both surveys respondents were asked "how is your health generally". The response categories were "Excellent", "Good", "Fair" and "Poor" at ages 23, 33, 42 and 44 in the 1958 cohort, as well as at ages 26 and

30 in the 1970 cohort. At age 46 in the 1958 cohort the response format was altered slightly with "very poor" added as a category. At ages 50 and 55 the response was altered to "Excellent", Very Good", "Good", "Fair" and "Poor". An identical format to this was used at ages 34, 38 and 42 in the 1970 cohort. In order to equalise the response format to a 5 point scale for all waves of both cohorts we employed the linear stretch method (de Jonge, Veenhoven, & Arends, 2014). For ease of interpretation all items were treated as continuous with a high scores representing poor health. We also performed sensitivity analysis using a binary version of the self-rated health. The derived binary item distinguished those who reported excellent health with all other participants. The response category "Excellent" appears in an identical format in all waves of both cohorts.

4.2.3 Statistical Modelling

We employed Latent Growth Models (LGM) where the repeated self-rated health measures are indicators for latent growth factors values for each individual. The latent growth model specification can be thought of as a Confirmatory Factor Analytic model and is a restricted form of a more general structural equation model (SEM; Kline 2010). In this formulation of a latent growth model, there are T repeated measures that serve as the indicators or manifest variables, self-rated health in this instance, where T is the number of time points or waves during which study participants were assessed. For a linear latent growth curve model, there are two latent factors: an intercept and a slope. The intercept captures the starting point of and individual variation around this, whereas the slope captures the average change over time and individual variation around the mean trend. Non linearities in the trends were captured with a flexible specification of LGMs where in between time points were not fixed but were freely estimated (Bollen & Curran, 2006).

$$\mathrm{SRHt}_t^C = \mathrm{i}_i + \mathrm{s}_i\ \mathrm{time}_{ti} + \varepsilon_{ti} \quad (4.1)$$

In Eq. 4.1 SRHt_t^C refers to a measure of the cohort member's Self Rated Health (SRH) at time t, i_i to a random intercept or the SRH level at baseline (age 23 on NCDSA and 26 on BCS70), s_i is a random slope that captures the average change in SRH over time. Typically, for the available sweeps (1) expands to a system of linear equations from which I and S are estimated given the measured SRH scores and time. The association between Year of Birth (YoB—1958 vs. 1970) and self-rated health at specific ages was modelled with linear regression:

$$\mathrm{SRH} = \alpha_1 + \beta_1.\mathrm{YoB} + \varepsilon_1 \quad (4.2)$$

We estimated the LGMs with Full Information Maximum Likelihood (FIML), a principled approach for missing data handling that operates under the Missing At

Random (MAR) assumption. It is widely accepted that under MAR, FIML returns unbiased estimates in the presence of missing data (Enders, 2001; Little & Rubin, 1989, 2002). The basic goal of FIML is to identify the population parameter values that are most likely to have produced a particular sample of data. In this context the MAR assumption implies that the occurrence of missing data depends on variables which are included in the model. Taking into account the well-known differences between men and women with respect to mortality rates (Pongiglione, De Stavola, Kuper, & Ploubidis, 2016) we present results stratified by gender. All our models were estimated with Mplus 7.4 (Muthen & Muthen, 1998–2015) with the Robust Maximum Likelihood (MLR) estimator with Monte Carlo integration (200 integration points).

4.3 Results

In Graphs 4.2a and 4.2b we present period life expectancy for both cohorts at various ages of the life course. In all ages and for both men and women those born in 1970 are expected to live two to three years longer on average. Confirming international trends, women were expected to live on average three to four years longer than men in all stages of the life course up to age 60. In Table 4.1 we present the means and 95% confidence intervals of self-rated health for men and women in the two cohorts. Despite expected to live longer, men and women born in 1970 reported similar self-rated health with those born in 1958 up to age 34, but worse self-rated health in midlife (age 42). As expected from the reported means and 95% confidence intervals, at age 33 the difference between the two cohorts was not significant, neither in men b = −0.007, 95% CI (−0.004 to 0.027) or women b = 0.002, 95% CI (−0.016 to 0.021). On the contrary, at age 42 the men and women born in 1970 reported significantly worse self-rated health compared to men and women born in 1958, with b = 0.324, 95% CI (0.284 to 0.363) in men and b = 0.118, 95% CI (0.100 to 0.136) in women (results differ slightly from raw means as missing data are taken into account in the reported linear regression coefficients). As it can be seen in Graph 4.3, as both cohorts age, they report worse self-rated health, but whereas in the 1958 cohort where with the exception of a "bump" at age 46, which is likely die to a mode effect since this survey was conducted via telephone, the trend is almost linear, whereas in the 1970 cohort both men and women report similar self-rated health up to age 34, and increasingly worse self-rated health at ages 38 and 42.

In Table 4.2 we present LGM parameters. As expected from the descriptive statistics the mean slope was of similar magnitude, positive and significant in both cohorts for both genders. With respect to the variance, there was significant variation around the intercept in both cohorts, which almost doubled in women born in 1970. There was some variation round the average slope in the 1958 cohort in both men and women indicating a degree of heterogeneity around the average population trajectory of self-rated health. On the contrary the estimated slope variance in both men and

Table 4.1 Mean self-rated health and 95% confidence intervals

1958 Cohort	Men				Women			
	n	Mean	95% CI		n	Mean	95% CI	
Age23—1981	6258	1.707	1.685	1.729	6266	1.826	1.804	1.849
Age33—1991	5548	1.942	1.918	1.967	5727	1.995	1.970	2.019
Age42—2000	5601	2.098	2.072	2.125	5773	2.126	2.099	2.152
Age44—2002	4523	2.272	2.247	2.297	4591	2.287	2.262	2.312
Age46—2004	4642	1.979	1.953	2.005	4885	2.044	2.017	2.071
Age50—2008	4784	2.520	2.489	2.551	4949	2.528	2.497	2.559
Age55—2013	4379	2.622	2.591	2.653	4660	2.675	2.644	2.706
1970 Cohort	Men				Women			
	n	Mean	95% CI		n	Mean	95% CI	
Age26—1986	4067	1.850	1.823	1.877	4856	1.930	1.906	1.954
Age30—2000	5416	2.034	2.008	2.059	5743	2.015	1.990	2.039
Age34—2004	4589	1.924	1.900	1.949	5009	1.990	1.964	2.015
Age38—2008	4170	2.292	2.262	2.322	4629	2.260	2.230	2.289
Age42—2012	4680	2.420	2.390	2.451	5068	2.378	2.348	2.408

women born in 1970 was minimal, indicating a relatively homogeneous evolution of self-rated health over the life course.

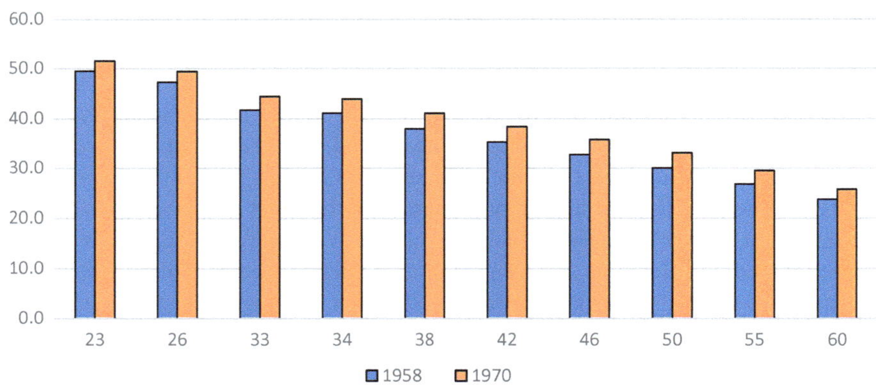

Graph 4.2a Period Life Expectancy in adulthood in the 1958 and 1970 cohorts—Men

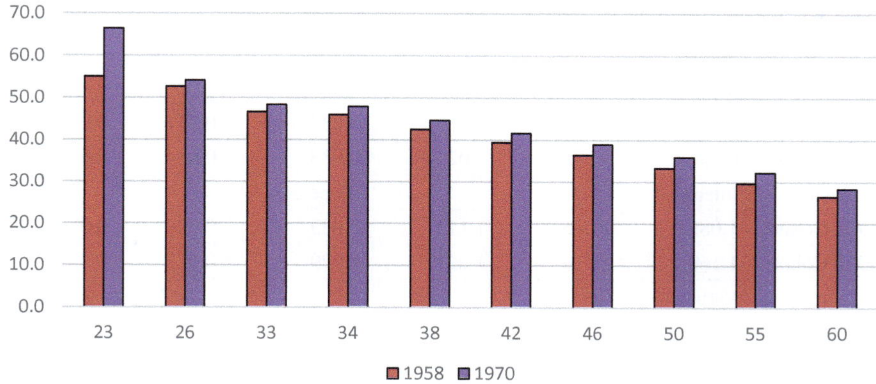

Graph 4.2b Period Life Expectancy in adulthood in the 1958 and 1970 cohorts—Women

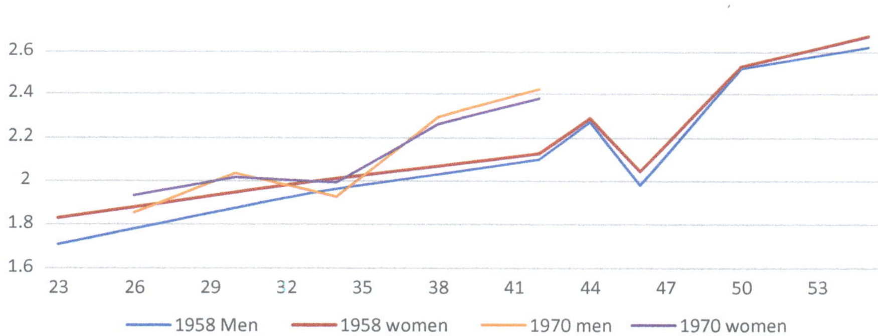

Graph 4.3 Mean self rated health in adulthood in the 1958 and 1970 cohorts—high score indicates poor health

4.4 Discussion

Mortality rates and life expectancy have traditionally been used as indicators of population health, but with the completion of the "epidemiological transition" in high and low-and-middle income countries (Omran, 2005), mortality has ceased to be as linked to health, and life expectancy does no longer fully capture the health status of a population. Studies that consider the joint progress of health and mortality are therefore needed. In this chapter we investigated the progress of self-rated health over the life course in two well characterised population based representative birth cohort studies in Britain. The two cohorts have experienced different mortality rates, which were lower in the more recently born cohort (those born in 1970). The evolution of self-rated health over time differed between the two cohorts, both with respect to the shape of change over time as well as the average level of reported self-rated health.

Table 4.2 Latent growth model parameters and 95% confidence intervals

	Mean					
Men	Intercept			Slope		
1958 Cohort	0.930	0.894	0.965	0.032	0.031	0.033
1970 Cohort	0.958	0.892	1.024	0.036	0.034	0.038
Women	Intercept			Slope		
1958 Cohort	1.082	1.046	1.113	0.029	0.028	0.030
1970 Cohort	1.169	1.110	1.227	0.029	0.027	0.031
	Variance					
Men	Intercept			Slope		
1958 Cohort	0.506	0.400	0.613	0.002	0.001	0.003
1970 Cohort	0.603	0.392	0.875	0.001	0.001	0.001
Women	Intercept			Slope		
1958 Cohort	0.530	0.425	0.635	0.001	−0.001	0.002
1970 Cohort	1.024	0.755	1.292	0.001	0.001	0.001

In the earlier born 1958 cohort—perhaps as expected—self rated health exhibited an almost linear trend with increasingly worse self-rated health being reported by both men and women as they moved from early adulthood to early old age. A different pattern was observed in the later born 1970 cohort, where the average level of self-rated health remained stable up to age 34, but steadily declined from age 38 onwards in both men and women. Despite the different trends, in both cohorts substantial variation was observed in the starting point of self-rated health, whereas on the contrary the evolution of self-rated health over time was relatively homogenous.

In both men and women, the two cohorts reported similar level of self-rated health in early adulthood, but the trend diverged at age 42, where the 1970 cohort reported their health being significantly worse. This observation is in accordance with recent findings on obesity and psychological distress where the more recently born cohorts were found to be more likely to be obese or overweight at stages of the life course (Johnson, Li, Kuh, & Hardy, 2015) and also experience more symptoms of psychological distress in midlife (Ploubidis, Sullivan, Brown, & Goodman, 2017). On the other hand, our findings do not agree with those from studies in the older population of the UK where the compression of morbidity hypothesis was supported for severe, but not mild disability (Jagger et al., 2016). The observation that the 1970 cohort report similar and eventually worse self-rated compared to an earlier born cohort in midlife has implications for public health policy in the UK. Taking into account that due to increases in life expectancy younger (more recently born) cohorts are expected to live longer, a necessary condition for compression of morbidity—in order for the added years to be lived healthily—is that controlling for age differences (or at a fixed age as in our paper), more recently born cohorts are healthier, so the average onset of morbidity is postponed (Fries, 1980; Fries et al., 2011). Our observation of similar up to age 34 and then worse average self-rated health in the

1970 cohort increases the likelihood of expansion of morbidity, assuming that the observed difference as well as the lower mortality rates in the 1970 cohort will persist in the future. Therefore, unless as both cohorts age, those born in 1958 catch up and surpass the 1970 cohort on average levels of self-rated health, our findings imply that the average onset of morbidity will not be postponed in the 1970 cohort.

Our results confirmed the well-established gender paradox with respect to health and mortality, which was first observed in the mid-1970s (Nathanson, 1975) and reflects the finding that women live longer than men, but tend to have worse health and more disability. Many theories have been proposed to explain the 'gender paradox' in mortality and disability, among which the most prevalent is that women may have higher prevalence of nonfatal but disabling diseases and men have higher prevalence of fatal and chronic diseases strongly related to mortality, whereas other hypothesise that the worse average health among women reflects their longer survival with ill health and/or disability, rather than just higher incidence of poor health, disability or chronic conditions (Pongiglione et al., 2016). In both cohorts, women experienced lower mortality rates and were thus expected to live longer than men, but they also reported similar self-rated health in all stages of the life course that were considered in this study. To the best of our knowledge, this is one of the few studies which show that the origin of the gender paradox—at least in Britain—may lie in early adulthood and midlife. The fact that self-rated health captures both non-fatal, but disabling diseases, as well as chronic diseases strongly related to mortality, does not allow us to interpret our findings in favour of any of the proposed theories. We note however, that in both cohorts women are likely to spend more years with poor or very poor self-rated health since they are expected to live longer, which indicates that the gender paradox at least in the two cohorts we considered in our study may be due to women's longer future survival despite poor/not good health.

Strengths of this study are the availability of two representative population based birth cohorts with self-rated health assessments at the same stages of the life-course and our analytic strategy which allowed us to capture intergenerational differences in the evolution of self-rated heath over time. Limitations include our reliance on self-reported data. Despite our efforts equalising the self-rated health items, random or systematic measurement error could have influenced our findings. Despite its widespread use in the quest for an indicator of "true" population health status (Quesnel-Vallee, 2007) and the agreement that this simple global question provides a useful summary of how people perceive their overall health status (Fayers & Sprangers, 2002), self-rated health is not without its limitations. In common with other self-reported measures, it suffers from the influence of response bias, such as social desirability (Hebert et al., 2001) and it has also been shown that the information people use to assess their own health is derived from a combination of information about specific health problems, general physical functioning, health behaviours (Benyamini, Leventhal, & Leventhal, 2003; Krause & Jay, 1994), mental health (Singh-Manoux et al., 2006), their genetic propensity to many common psychiatric and physical disorders as well as psychological traits (Harris et al., 2016), as well as general social experience (Sen, 2002). It is likely that the weight individuals assign to these health domains when assessing their overall health status varies and evidence shows that, for example, there may be differences in the way which individuals of high and low socioeconomic position assess their health (Dowd & Zajacova, 2007), in addition to differences between men and women (Benyamini, Blumstein, Lusky, & Modan, 2003), differences between national populations (Desesquelles, Egidi, & Salvatore, 2009) and differences between age groups (Singh-Manoux et al., 2007).

Differences in reporting styles between generations are therefore possible and they may have contributed to the observed between cohort variation. Having only one item available to capture self-rated health did allow us to embark on formal measurement invariance testing between the cohorts (Ploubidis et al., 2017). However, we have recently shown that strong/metric measurement invariance can be obtained in self-reports of psychological distress (Ploubidis et al., 2017). This implies that the passage of 12 years hasn't differentially affected the interpretation of the survey questions that tap into symptoms of psychological distress and we believe it's reasonable to assume that same holds for self-rated health. Sensitivity analysis employing an identical binary version of self-rated health in both cohorts that distinguished those in "excellent" health from others returned very similar results reinforcing our interpretation that the differences in the format of the self-rated health item in the two cohorts did not bias our results. Another limitation is that we assumed an identical missing data generating mechanism in both cohorts, which implies that an identical set of observed variables are responsible for the occurrence of missing data in both studies. It should also be noted that the 1970 cohort had a higher prevalence of missing data in the self-rated health items. We report estimates allowing only a small fraction of missing data in the outcome in our models, and note that similar results were obtained in analyses with varying missing data inclusion criteria, including imputation of all missing data in the self-rated health outcomes.

Our results showcase the association between year of birth and self-rated health, but our analysis could not disentangle whether the observed difference is due to "cohort" or "period" effects (Keyes, Utz, Robinson, & Li, 2010). It is well known that Age—Period—Cohort models cannot be identified without added constraints, since no statistical model can simultaneously estimate age, period, and cohort effects because of the collinearity among these variables (Keyes et al., 2010). We note that establishing the age adjusted association between year of birth and self-rated health is sufficient as an empirical test of compression of morbidity. Understanding whether the association between year of birth and self-rated health is due to "cohort" or "period" effects is a further step beyond the scope of this paper, which under assumptions would provide us with valuable insights on the mechanism that underlies the observed association between year of birth and psychological distress.

The observed increase in the reporting of worse self-rated health experienced by the 1970 cohort in mid-life in Britain has policy implications, given that the increase has occurred despite economic growth. The 1958 cohort are part of the 'Lucky Generation' of post-war baby boomers, who experienced high absolute levels of social mobility, and lower levels of social inequality, whereas the 1970 cohort are part of 'Generation X', who have experienced greater uncertainty and insecurity over the whole of their adult lives and a more individualistic ideological climate (Sullivan, Brown, & Bann, 2015). If these generational changes lie behind the average worse self-rated health of the 1970 cohort, then we would predict that future generations will be worse off still if such trends were to continue. A better understanding of the aetiological mechanism that underlies twill open up possibilities for ways to promote healthy ageing and has the potential to inform policy making and future population based interventions. Future work employing more cohorts, such as the 1946 and Millennium cohort studies, in order to test whether the observed health disadvantage of the more recently born cohort represents a general trend is warranted. Ideally this work should employ more health outcomes, especially observe measured health indicators that have been linked with specific chronic diseases, as well as various disability indicators. This will be a first step in understanding the mechanism that underlies the worsening of self-rated health in the 1970 cohort and whether this is mostly due to the recently documented mental health disadvantage of the 1970 cohort in midlife or other health conditions are also responsible. Employing a wide range of health indicators over different stages of the life course will also provide an empirical test of the two competing theories with respect to the gender paradox.

Further analysis of the British birth cohorts as they move towards old age will also provide insights on the underlying mechanism of the worsening of self-rated health in those born in 1970. For example a recent study of the older population in the UK (Jagger et al., 2016) found that mild disability is expanding whereas severe disability is compressing. Further work is needed to investigate whether the worsening of self-rated health of more recently born cohorts in the working age population of the UK will replicate the disability trends observed in the older population as the current working age cohorts move towards old age. Furthermore, considering that it's not possible to calculate healthy life expectancy estimates for a particular age within a single cohort without very strong assumptions, an individual level quantity that captures years spend with ill health, a particular chronic condition and/or disability, that also combines morality information within each cohort would be a very welcome addition to this line of work. Finally, the abundance of information available in the UK birth cohorts will allow the investigation of the underlying mechanism of expansion, as for example in a recent study (Ploubidis et al., 2017) where it was shown that early life characteristics only modestly account for the increasing level of midlife psychological distress in more recently born cohorts.

References

Bebbington, A. C., & Darton, R. A. (1996). *Healthy Life Expectancy in England and Wales: Recent Evidence*. Retrieved from Personal Social Services Research Unit.

Benyamini, Y., Blumstein, T., Lusky, A., & Modan, B. (2003a). Gender differences in the self-rated health-mortality association: Is it poor self-rated health that predicts mortality or excellent self-rated health that predicts survival? *Gerontologist, 43*(3), 396–405.

Benyamini, Y., Leventhal, E. A., & Leventhal, H. (2003b). Elderly people's ratings of the importance of health-related factors to their self-assessments of health. *Social Science and Medicine, 56*(8), 1661–1667.

Birnie, K., Ben-Shlomo, Y., Gunnell, D., Ebrahim, S., Bayer, A., Gallacher, J., & Martin, R. M. (2011). Diet in childhood and adulthood and physical performance in old age: Findings from the Boyd Orr and Caerphilly cohorts. *Journal of Epidemiology and Community Health, 65*. https://doi.org/10.1136/jech.2011.143586.77.

Birnie, K., Cooper, R., Martin, R. M., Kuh, D., Sayer, A. A., Alvarado, B. E., ... Team, H. A. S. (2011). Childhood socioeconomic position and objectively measured physical capability levels in adulthood: A systematic review and meta-analysis. *Plos One, 6*(1), e15564. https://doi.org/10.1371/journal.pone.0015564.

Bollen, K. A., & Curran, P. J. (2006). *Latent curve models: A structural equation perspective* (Vol. 467). New York: Wiley.

Bowling, A. (1995). *Measuring disease: A handbook for the assessment of quality of life*. Milton Keynes: Open University Press.

Cambois, E., Robine, J. M., & Hayward, M. D. (2001). Social inequalities in disability-free life expectancy in the french male population, 1980–1991. *Demography, 38*(4), 513–524. https://doi.org/10.1353/dem.2001.0033.

Cooper, R., Strand, B. H., Hardy, R., Patel, K. V., & Kuh, D. (2014). *Physical capability in mid-life and survival over 13 years of follow-up: British birth cohort study* (Vol. 348).

Crimmins, E. M., & Beltran-Sanchez, H. (2011). Mortality and morbidity trends: is there compression of morbidity? *Journals of Gerontology Series B-Psychological Sciences and Social Sciences, 66*(1), 75–86. https://doi.org/10.1093/geronb/gbq088.

Crimmins, E. M., Saito, Y., & Ingegneri, D. (1997). Trends in disability-free life expectancy in the United States, 1970–1990. *Population and Development Review, 23*(3), 555- + . https://doi.org/10.2307/2137572.

Crimmins, E. M., Saito, Y., & Kim, J. K. (2016a). Change in cognitively healthy and cognitively impaired life expectancy in the United States: 2000–2010. *SSM Population Health, 2*, 793–797. https://doi.org/10.1016/j.ssmph.2016.10.007.

Crimmins, E. M., Zhang, Y., & Saito, Y. (2016b). Trends over 4 decades in disability-free life expectancy in the United States. *American Journal of Public Health, 106*(7), 1287–1293. https://doi.org/10.2105/ajph.2016.303120.

de Jonge, T., Veenhoven, R., & Arends, L. (2014). Homogenizing responses to different survey questions on the same topic: Proposal of a scale homogenization method using a reference distribution. *Social Indicators Research, 117*(1), 275–300. https://doi.org/10.1007/s11205-013-0335-6.

DeSalvo, K. B., Bloser, N., Reynolds, K., He, J., & Muntner, P. (2006). Mortality prediction with a single general self-rated health question. *Journal of General Internal Medicine, 21*(3), 267–275.

Desesquelles, A. F., Egidi, V., & Salvatore, M. A. (2009). Why do Italian people rate their health worse than French people do? An exploration of cross-country differentials of self-rated health. *Social Science and Medicine, 68*(6), 1124–1128.

Dowd, J. B., & Zajacova, A. (2007). Does the predictive power of self-rated health for subsequent mortality risk vary by socioeconomic status in the US? *International Journal of Epidemiology, 36*, 1214–1221. https://doi.org/10.1093/ije/dym214lISSN0300-5771.

Enders, C. K. (2001). The performance of the full information maximum likelihood estimator in multiple regression models with missing data. *Educational and Psychological Measurement, 61*(5), 713–740. https://doi.org/10.1177/0013164401615001.

Fayers, P. M., & Sprangers, M. A. G. (2002). Understanding self-rated health. *Lancet, 359*(9302), 187–188.

Fries, J. F. (1980). Aging, natural death, and the compression of morbidity. *New England Journal of Medicine, 303*(3), 130–135. https://doi.org/10.1056/nejm198007173030304.

Fries, J. F. (1996). Physical activity, the compression of morbidity, and the health of the elderly. *Journal of the Royal Society of Medicine, 89*(2), 64–68.

Fries, J. F. (2005). Frailty, heart disease, and stroke: The compression of morbidity paradigm. *American Journal of Preventive Medicine, 29*(5, Supplement 1), 164–168. http://dx.doi.org/10.1016/j.amepre.2005.07.004.

Fries, J. F., Bruce, B., & Chakravarty, E. (2011). Compression of morbidity 1980–2011: a focused review of paradigms and progress. *Journal of Aging Research, 2011*, 261702–261702. https://doi.org/10.4061/2011/261702.

Giele, J. Z., & Elder, G. H. (1998). *Methods of life course research: qualitative and quantitative approaches*. Thousand Oaks: Sage Publications.

Gruenberg, E. M. (1977). Failures of success. *Milbank Memorial Fund Quarterly-Health and Society, 55*(1), 3–24. https://doi.org/10.2307/3349592.

Grundy, E., & Glaser, K. (2000). Socio-demographic differences in the onset and progression of disability in early old age: A longitudinal study. *Age and Ageing, 29*(2), 149–157.

Harris, S. E., Hagenaars, S. P., Davies, G., Hill, W. D., Liewald, D. C., Ritchie, S. J., … McIntosh, A. M. (2016). Molecular genetic contributions to self-rated health. *International Journal of Epidemiology*, dyw219.

Hebert, J. R., Peterson, K. E., Hurley, T. G., Stoddard, A. M., Cohen, N., Field, A. E., & Sorensen, G. (2001). The effect of social desirability trait on self-reported dietary measures among multi-ethnic female health center employees. *Annals of Epidemiology, 11*(6), 417–427.

Hessler, R. M., Eriksson, B. G., Dey, D., Steen, G., Sundh, V., & Steen, B. (2003). The compression of morbidity debate in aging: an empirical test using the gerontological and geriatric population studies in Göteborg, Sweden (H70). *Archives of Gerontology and Geriatrics, 37*(3), 213–222. https://doi.org/10.1016/S0167-4943(03)00048-7.

Hubert, H. B., Bloch, D. A., Oehlert, J. W., & Fries, J. F. (2002). Lifestyle habits and compression of morbidity. *The Journals of Gerontology Series A: Biological Sciences and Medical Sciences, 57*(6), M347–M351. https://doi.org/10.1093/gerona/57.6.M347.

Human Mortality Database. (2015). Retrieved February 2, 2015, from www.mortality.org or www.humanmortality.de.

Idler, E. L., & Benyamini, Y. (1997). Self-rated health and mortality: A review of twenty-seven community studies. *Journal of Health and Social Behavior, 38*(1), 21–37.

Jagger, C., Matthews, F. E., Wohland, P., Fouweather, T., Stephan, B. C., Robinson, L., … Brayne, C. (2016). A comparison of health expectancies over two decades in England: Results of the cognitive function and ageing study I and II. *Lancet, 387*(10020), 779–786. https://doi.org/10.1016/s0140-6736(15)00947-2.

Jagger, C., Matthews, F. E., Wohland, P., Fouweather, T., Stephan, B. C. M., Robinson, L., … Brayne, C. (2017). A comparison of health expectancies over two decades in England: Results of the cognitive function and ageing study I and II. *The Lancet, 387*(10020), 779–786. https://doi.org/10.1016/s0140-6736(15)00947-2.

Johnson, W., Li, L., Kuh, D., & Hardy, R. (2015). How has the age-related process of overweight or obesity development changed over time? Co-ordinated analyses of individual participant data from five United Kingdom birth cohorts. *Plos Medicine, 12*(5), e1001828. https://doi.org/10.1371/journal.pmed.1001828.

Keyes, K. M., Utz, R. L., Robinson, W., & Li, G. (2010). What is a cohort effect? Comparison of three statistical methods for modeling cohort effects in obesity prevalence in the United States, 1971–2006. *Social Science and Medicine, 70*(7), 1100–1108. https://doi.org/10.1016/j.socscimed.2009.12.018.

Khaw, K. T. (1997). Healthy aging. *British Medical Journal, 315*(7115), 1090–1096.

Krause, N. M., & Jay, G. M. (1994). What do global self-rated health items measure. *Medical Care, 32*(9), 930–942.

Kuh, D., & Ben-Shlomo, Y. (2004). *A life course approach to chronic disease epidemiology*: Oxford: Oxford University Press.

Kuh, D., Ben-Shlomo, Y., Lynch, J., Hallqvist, J., & Power, C. (2003). Life course epidemiology. *Journal of Epidemiology and Community Health, 57*(10), 778–783. https://doi.org/10.1136/jech.57.10.778.

Leon, D. A. (2011). Trends in european life expectancy: a salutary view. *International Journal of Epidemiology, 40*(2), 271–277. https://doi.org/10.1093/ije/dyr061.

Leon, D. A., Lithell, H. O., Vagero, D., Koupilova, I., Mohsen, R., Berglund, L., ... McKeigue, P. M. (1998). Reduced fetal growth rate and increased risk of death from ischaemic heart disease: cohort study of 15 000 Swedish men and women born 1915–1929. *British Medical Journal, 317*(7153), 241–245.

Little, R. J. A., & Rubin, D. B. (1989). The analysis of social-science data with missing values. *Sociological Methods & Research, 18*(2–3), 292–326.

Little, R. J. A., & Rubin, D. B. (2002). *Statistical analysis with missing data* (2nd ed.). Chichester: Wiley.

Mackenbach, J. P., & Looman, C. W. (2013). Life expectancy and national income in Europe, 1900–2008: an update of Preston's analysis. *International Journal of Epidemiology*. https://doi.org/10.1093/ije/dyt122.

Manton, K. G. (1982). Changing concepts of morbidity and mortality in the elderly population. *Milbank Memorial Fund Quarterly-Health and Society, 60*(2), 183–244. https://doi.org/10.2307/3349767.

Manton, K. G. (2008). Recent declines in chronic disability in the elderly US population: Risk factors and future dynamics. *Annual Review of Public Health, 29,* 91–113.

Manton, K. G., Stallard, E., & Corder, L. S. (1998). The dynamics of dimensions of age-related disability 1982 to 1994 in the US elderly population. *Journals of Gerontology Series A-Biological Sciences and Medical Sciences, 53*(1), B59–B70.

Muthen, L. K., & Muthen, B. O. (1998–2015). *Mplus User's Guide. Seventh Edition*. Muthén & Muthén: Los Angeles.

Nathanson, C. A. (1975). Illness and the feminine role: a theoretical review. *Social Science and Medicine, 9*(2), 57–62.

Nusselder, W. J., Looman, C. W. N., van de Mheen, P. J. M., van de Mheen, H., & Mackenbach, J. P. (2000). Smoking and the compression of morbidity. *Journal of Epidemiology and Community Health, 54*(8), 566–574. https://doi.org/10.1136/jech.54.8.566.

Oeppen, J., & Vaupel, J. W. (2002). Demography - Broken limits to life expectancy. *Science, 296*(5570), 1029- + . https://doi.org/10.1126/science.1069675.

Olshansky, S. J., Rudberg, M. A., Carnes, B. A., Cassel, C. K., & Brody, J. A. (1991). Trading off longer life for worsening health: The expansion of morbidity hypothesis. *Journal of Aging and Health, 3*(2), 194–216. https://doi.org/10.1177/089826439100300205.

Omran, A. R. (1971). Epidemiologic transition - theory of epidemiology of population change. *Milbank Memorial Fund Quarterly, 49*(4), 509-&. https://doi.org/10.2307/3349375.

Omran, A. R. (2005). The epidemiologic transition: A theory of the epidemiology of population change. *Milbank Quarterly, 83*(4), 731–757. https://doi.org/10.1111/j.1468-0009.2005.00398.x.

Peres, K., Jagger, C., Matthews, F. E., & Mrc, C. (2008). Impact of late-life self-reported emotional problems on disability-free life expectancy: Results from the MRC cognitive function and ageing study. *International Journal of Geriatric Psychiatry, 23*(6), 643–649. https://doi.org/10.1002/gps.1955.

Ploubidis, G. B., Sullivan, A., Brown, M., & Goodman, A. (2017). Psychological distress in mid-life: evidence from the 1958 and 1970 British birth cohorts. *Psychological Medicine, 47*(2), 291–303. https://doi.org/10.1017/s0033291716002464.

Polder, J. J., Barendregt, J. J., & van Oers, H. (2006). Health care costs in the last year of life - the Dutch experience. *Social Science and Medicine, 63*(7), 1720–1731. https://doi.org/10.1016/j.socscimed.2006.04.018.

Pongiglione, B., De Stavola, B. L., Kuper, H., & Ploubidis, G. B. (2016). Disability and all-cause mortality in the older population: Evidence from the english longitudinal study of ageing. *European Journal of Epidemiology, 31*(8), 735–746. https://doi.org/10.1007/s10654-016-0160-8.

Power, C., & Elliott, J. (2006). Cohort profile: 1958 British birth cohort (national child development study). *International Journal of Epidemiology, 35*(1), 34–41. https://doi.org/10.1093/ije/dyi183.

Quesnel-Vallee, A. (2007). Self-rated health: Caught in the crossfire of the quest for 'true' health? *International Journal of Epidemiology, 36*(6), 1161–1164.

Robine, J. M., & Mathers, C. M. (1993). Measuring the compression or expansion of morbidity through changes in health expectancy. In J. M. Robine (Ed.), *Calculation of health expectancies, harmonization, consensus achieved and future perspectives* (pp. 169–286). Paris: Libbey.

Robine, J.-M., Romieu, I., & Cambois, E. (1999). Health expectancy indicators. *Bulletin-World Health Organization, 77,* 181–185.

Salomon, J. A., Wang, H., Freeman, M. K., Vos, T., Flaxman, A. D., Lopez, A. D., & Murray, C. J. L. (2012). Healthy life expectancy for 187 countries, 1990–2010: A systematic analysis for the global burden disease study 2010. *The Lancet, 380*(9859), 2144–2162. http://dx.doi.org/10.1016/S0140-6736(12)61690-0.

Sen, A. (2002). Health: perception versus observation - self reported morbidity has severe limitations and can be extremely misleading. *British Medical Journal, 324*(7342), 860–861.

Singh-Manoux, A., Dugravot, A., Shipley, M. J., Ferrie, J., Martikainen, P., Goldberg, M., & Zins, M. (2007). The association between self-rated health and mortality in different socioeconomic groups in the GAZEL cohort study. *International Journal of Epidemiology, 36,* 1222–1228.

Singh-Manoux, A., Martikainen, P., Ferrie, J., Zins, M., Marmot, M., & Goldberg, M. (2006). What does self rated health measure? Results from the British Whitehall II and French Gazel cohort studies. *Journal of Epidemiology and Community Health, 60*(4), 364–372.

Sullivan, A., Brown, M., & Bann, D. (2015). Guest editorial: Generation X enters middle age. *Longitudinal and Life Course Studies, 6*(2), 120–130.

van de Water, H. P. A., Boshuizen, H. C., & Perenboom, R. J. M. (1996). *Health expectancy in the Netherlands 1983–1990* (Vol. 6).

Waidmann, T., Bound, J., & Schoenbaum, M. (1995). The illusion of failure - trends in the self reported health of the US elderly. *Milbank Quarterly, 73*(2), 253–287. https://doi.org/10.2307/3350259.

Waynforth, D. (2012). Grandparental investment and reproductive decisions in the longitudinal 1970 British cohort study. *Proceedings of the Royal Society B-Biological Sciences, 279*(1731), 1155–1160. https://doi.org/10.1098/rspb.2011.1424.

Werblow, A., Felder, S., & Zweifel, P. (2007). Population ageing and health care expenditure: A school of 'red herrings'? *Health Economics, 16*(10), 1109–1126. https://doi.org/10.1002/hec.1213.

Yong, V., & Saito, Y. (2009). Trends in healthy life expectancy in Japan: 1986–2004. *Demographic Research, 20,* 467–494.

Zweifel, P., Felder, S., & Meiers, M. (1999). Ageing of population and health care expenditure: A red herring? *Health Economics, 8*(6), 485–496. https://doi.org/10.1002/(sici)1099-1050(199909)8:6%3c485:aid-hec461%3e3.0.co;2-4.

MIX
Papier aus verantwortungsvollen Quellen
Paper from responsible sources
FSC® C105338

If you have any concerns about our products,
you can contact us on
ProductSafety@springernature.com

In case Publisher is established outside the EU,
the EU authorized representative is:
Springer Nature Customer Service Center GmbH
Europaplatz 3, 69115 Heidelberg, Germany

Printed by Libri Plureos GmbH
in Hamburg, Germany